Menopause the D

Dr Juliet Bressan is a public health doctor and GP, and the author of hundreds of articles on women's health and well-being. In addition to having published several books, she is a resident television doctor with Ireland's independent television channel TV3. Dr Bressan lives in Dublin with her husband and two grown-up daughters. For more information, go to www.julietbressan.com.

Overcoming Common Problems Series

Selected titles

A full list of titles is available from Sheldon Press,
36 Causton Street, London SW1P 4ST and on our website at
www.sheldonpress.co.uk

101 Questions to Ask Your Doctor
Dr Tom Smith

Asperger Syndrome in Adults
Dr Ruth Searle

The Assertiveness Handbook
Mary Hartley

Assertiveness: Step by step
Dr Windy Dryden and Daniel Constantinou

Backache: What you need to know
Dr David Delvin

Birth Over 35
Sheila Kitzinger

Body Language: What you need to know
David Cohen

Bulimia, Binge-eating and their Treatment
Professor J. Hubert Lacey, Dr Bryony Bamford
and Amy Brown

The Cancer Survivor's Handbook
Dr Terry Priestman

The Chronic Pain Diet Book
Neville Shone

Cider Vinegar
Margaret Hills

Coeliac Disease: What you need to know
Alex Gazzola

Coping Successfully with Pain
Neville Shone

Coping Successfully with Prostate Cancer
Dr Tom Smith

Coping Successfully with Shyness
Margaret Oakes, Professor Robert Bor
Dr Carina Eriksen

Coping Successfully with Ulcerative Colitis
Peter Cartwright

Coping Successfully with Varicose Veins
Christine Craggs-Hinton

Coping Successfully with Your Hiatus Hernia
Dr Tom Smith

Coping Successfully with Your Irritable Bowel
Rosemary Nicol

Coping When Your Child Has Cerebral Palsy
Jill Eckersley

Coping with Anaemia
Dr Tom Smith

Coping with Asthma in Adults
Mark Greener

Coping with Birth Trauma and Postnatal Depression
Lucy Jolin

Coping with Bowel Cancer
Dr Tom Smith

Coping with Bronchitis and Emphysema
Dr Tom Smith

Coping with Candida
Shirley Trickett

Coping with Chemotherapy
Dr Terry Priestman

Coping with Chronic Fatigue
Trudie Chalder

Coping with Coeliac Disease
Karen Brody

Coping with Diverticulitis
Peter Cartwright

Coping with Drug Problems in the Family
Lucy Jolin

Coping with Dyspraxia
Jill Eckersley

Coping with Early-onset Dementia
Jill Eckersley

Coping with Eating Disorders and Body Image
Christine Craggs-Hinton

Coping with Envy
Dr Windy Dryden

Coping with Gout
Christine Craggs-Hinton

Coping with Headaches and Migraine
Alison Frith

Coping with Heartburn and Reflux
Dr Tom Smith

Coping with Life after Stroke
Dr Mareeni Raymond

Coping with Life's Challenges: Moving on from adversity
Dr Windy Dryden

Overcoming Common Problems Series

Overcoming Common Problems Series

Overcoming Common Problems

Menopause
the Drug-free Way

DR JULIET BRESSAN

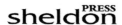
sheldon PRESS

First published in Great Britain in 2012

Sheldon Press
36 Causton Street
London SW1P 4ST
www.sheldonpress.co.uk

The author and publisher have made every effort to ensure that the external website and
email addresses included in this book are correct and up to date at the time of going to press.
The author and publisher are not responsible for the content, quality or continuing
accessibility of the sites.

The extract on p. 83 is from Billy Collins, 'Forgetfulness', *Sailing Alone Around the Room:
New and Selected Poems*, New York: Random House, 2002.

Every effort has been made to seek permission to use copyright material reproduced
in this book. The publisher apologizes for those cases where permission might not have been
sought and, if notified, will formally seek permission at the earliest opportunity.

British Library Cataloguing-in-Publication Data
A catalogue record for this book is available from the British Library

ISBN 978–1–84709–223–6
eBook ISBN 978–1–84709–224–3

Typeset by Caroline Waldron, Wirral, Cheshire
First printed in Great Britain by Ashford Colour Press
Subsequently digitally printed in Great Britain

eBook by Fakenham Photosetting Ltd, Fakenham, Norfolk

Produced on paper from sustainable forests

Contents

'Women will not keep under medical care for what they know to be a natural process.'

Diseases of Women, a Clinical Guide to their Diagnosis and Treatment, 1898

Introduction

For many decades, women were told by their doctors that the menopause was 'unnatural': doctors actually argued, very strongly, that women in 'nature' aren't supposed to live past 50. But then doctors also began to tell women that they didn't have to worry about hot flushes, tiredness, weight gain, depression, aches and pains, sleepless nights or wrinkles, because artificial hormones could take care of it all. And not only did artificial hormones after 50 make you feel better, younger, stronger, happier and healthier, they were going to protect your bones against fractures, improve your memory and give you back your much-lamented sex drive. Menopause, doctors reminded us, wasn't a natural condition to be in; the majority of us were supposed to die in childbirth, or shortly afterwards. But, in our 'unnatural', modern world, we have surprised the medical profession by surviving far past 50. No wonder we don't feel well!

And thankfully, doctors argued, the pharmaceutical industry can supply us with hormones to take care of all our needs. Therefore, we may live on, in this state of post-menopausal twilight, in an unnatural state of hormonal enhancement, despite the (then unknown) risks that that would bring.

Ever since the results of the Million Women Study were published at the end of the twentieth century, however, the medical profession have had to completely rethink their understanding of what they ought to 'do' about the menopause. The Million Women Study showed, irrefutably, that hormone replacement therapy, once the billion-dollar panacea of all female problems after 50, is firmly associated with cancer. It also proved that HRT does not actually protect bones, the heart or the mind. Since then, the medical profession has pretty much gone silent on how to manage this 'unnatural' situation of the woman who, defying nature, has had the nerve to live past 50, and often well into her eighties and nineties.

A baby girl born in 2007 in the UK currently has a life expectancy of 81.9 years. Life expectancy at age 65 – that is, the number of further years that someone reaching 65 in 2007–09 can expect to live – is much higher for women than for men. Based on current mortality rates, according to the Office for National Statistics, a woman aged 65 today can expect to live another 20.2 years. So it is perfectly natural for women in the twenty-first century to expect to finish with their fertility in the *middle* of their lives, to be followed by another 30 to 40 years of full, active, healthy post-menopausal life.

Our environment is quite 'unnatural'. Thanks to technological and industrial advances, we live long, active and productive lives. But we also live in an environment that is full of toxins and pollutants, both physical and emotional. We are exposed to all sorts of relationship stress and social turmoil, particularly in mid-life. We are challenged with having to embrace new technologies in our workplace, with the rapid expansion of cities, with ever more exhausting commutes, or with work-related foreign travel. In mid-life we may be faced with relationship breakdown, childcare stresses, teenage anxiety around drugs or even suicide, parental ill health – all of which can threaten every resource in our body and take a huge toll on our own life.

I believe, as a doctor and a woman, that we have to rethink completely our ideas about a 'natural' lifespan, and develop a more up-to-date understanding of where menopause and mid-life symptoms fit in. If we, as twenty-first-century women, are going to live for at least 85 years, and many of us longer, then 50 is genuinely only the middle of our productive lives. It isn't the 'end of fertility': it's the beginning of seniority. It's the gateway to real maturity. Just as puberty is the gateway to fertility – and oh, what a messy, unpleasant, troublesome time that seemed to be back then – menopause is the senior equivalent: a puberty for mature age. It's your body saying to you, quite unsympathetically: just when you thought that nothing would change for you in your self-satisfied, comfortable world, well, take a look at this then!

I want to put forward a strong, positive message about ageing in women, and that begins with the menopause. Just as many aspects of puberty do need medical evaluation (acne, depression, painful periods, uneven breast development, lack of personal confidence, sleep disorder, eating disorder), many of the changes that happen in our bodies during menopause need medical support. No woman can experience the menopause twice, so we are always going to be unprepared for the suddenness of the experience. However, despite the amount of coverage menopause gets in media and journalism,

I am always meeting, in the surgery, women who have begun to notice, in their forties, minor changes in their 'system' and ask me, very anxiously, if it could be menopause. In other words, despite all the hoo-ha that menopause provokes in both medical and mainstream media, the menopausal woman herself has no idea what to expect.

Irregular periods, absent periods, dry vagina, palpitations, low mood, painful bones – will it really be this bad? We think we know a lot about what it's going to be like – but the truth is that every woman's body is different, and the range of experiences is so diverse. Women worry because these symptoms can arrive suddenly, are uncomfortable, and interfere with daily life, with work, with social recreation, with motivation and energy. And we worry about the long-term effects of the loss of our fertility cycle, and how it will affect our relationship, our dreams and our desires. But most of all, we worry about how it will affect our ageing bodies and minds.

What if I develop osteoporosis, and end up with a hump on my back? What if I gain even more weight? What if my husband stops loving me because I can't bear to have sex any more? What if I get cancer – it's happened to so many of my friends? What if the loss of energy I feel becomes worse and I have to give up exercising or doing sport? What if this low mood is something more serious? How will I cope if I have a hot flush in the middle of that important job interview next week? These are very real, practical concerns that can't be dismissed by saying, 'Oh, the menopause is just a normal state of affairs, and you'll feel much better soon.'

We women in our forties and fifties are often at the height of our careers. We may be responsible for caring for two generations of dependants (children and elderly parents), and perhaps the only breadwinner in a family. Many of us are single parents. Some of us will have recently divorced. We may have only just had a baby, or may be parenting small toddlers. Many are caring for grandchildren. We need to feel strong, to feel empowered and to know that we can cope and protect our health from the new risks of long-term disease that we might otherwise face. We need to be able to ride the wave of bodily changes in mid-life and to maintain all the responsibilities that we already hold. We can't be expected to suffer in silence, or to take it on the chin.

But at the same time, we can't be fobbed off with pills and hormones any more. Today's menopausal woman needs a new roadmap; she wants to feel in control and to have the confidence to manage her own body, no matter what alarming symptoms it brings her. And she needs to look forward to old age, in the knowledge that she is, during her menopause, developing healthy, preventive, healing habits, so that her future years will be comfortable and disease-free.

What I want to do in this book is to go through the most important problems that menopause can raise for women, and to tease them out and suggest real solutions that work and that aren't just the dismissive product of an overactive prescription pad. I do believe (and, contrary to some of my colleagues in the heady days of mass-market HRT, I have always believed) that the menopause is a storm of bodily, mindful and spiritual transition in our journey into real growth and maturity. But I'm very, very aware that in our unforgiving, dynamic, exciting and modern world, the experience is full of really tough decisions, hideously unpleasant symptoms and scary health risks. Menopause will bring you problems if you aren't on top of it. The post-menopause years are a high-risk period for cancer, osteoporosis, dementia, heart disease, depression and stroke. If there's one positive message we should be getting when our periods cease, it is this. Stop. Look about you, at the world around you, and have a think. You are a mature woman now. You have a body that is becoming vulnerable in new ways, and you need to get to know how to treat it differently. Your body and your mind deserve a new respect.

Your bones, muscles, breasts, skin, teeth, eyes, bladder, digestive system, liver, heart and brain all need nourishing and protecting. And your mind, that wonderful, powerful place, which you previously took for granted to do all the hard work for you, now takes on a different, even more powerful role in your life. It needs cherishing, and in return it will bring you joy and comfort both now and later.

Growing older is inevitable, and although we can fight the external appearance with Botox and the gym, we have to experience, as women, the fact that the end of fertility changes our bodies for ever. There's no one-size-fits-all remedy that makes the menopause go away. Once fertility begins to fade, our new, post-fertile body needs to find its place in our self-awareness. This uncharted territory can be full of anxiety and distress, just as any uncertain journey into a very different way of thinking, feeling, working, eating, playing and loving has the potential to be. Or it can be an exciting and empowering journey of rejuvenation and self-discovery. It can be a time in which we use the new maturity we've gained to maximize our potential for total health and well-being through life, in a way in which we, as younger women, would never have had the wisdom to consider.

Fear of death is a pretty universal feeling. But why should we be afraid of becoming old? Ancient societies elevated the elderly, as their wiser, more important members, rather than hiding them away. But ancient societies were often full of spiritual, magical beliefs: superstition holds very little power in our modern, secular world. I've often thought that fear of death, in the absence of an innocent belief in the certainty of a magical, more powerful after-life, is what leads modern society to despise old age, to shrink from the wrinkles, to marginalize the elderly, to write them out of the story of life.

The menopause is a stark signal that the second half of our life has begun. We may be afraid that we're running out of time. The long, busy 'interval' of baby-making, career development, upward mobility and personal growth is moving into a new phase: we are slowing down. Old people don't appear attractive to us. We don't want to have to stop doing all the activities we love; we don't want to wear boring clothes or flat shoes. Just as the adolescent dreads the thought of growing up and having to get a job, we meno-pausal women see the grey hairs marching across our heads and we shudder to think what's going to happen next.

If you've picked up this book you are probably a woman in your late forties or early fifties. You may be a younger woman whose menopause has come prematurely, who doesn't want to turn to arti-ficial medicines that may affect you adversely in later life, or cause you side-effects. You may be a woman whose menopause has hap-pened very abruptly, as a result of cancer treatment or surgery to remove your ovaries, for example, for whom any sort of artificial hormone treatment is impossible, yet who desperately needs a solu-tion to the symptoms of menopause.

But if you have chosen this book among the many other meno-pause guides available, it's because you're looking for a drug-free way of managing your menopause. You may be tired of taking medicines. You may be sick of consulting your uninterested doctor. You probably want to know how you can stop feeling so unwell, so tired, so worried, and at the same time avoid expensive or potentially dangerous drugs.

You would probably like to take this period of change in your stride, to avoid the side-effects of pharmaceutical medicines, and at the same time get on top of all the difficult physical and emotional symptoms of menopause and live a long, happy, healthier life. And you want sound, well-researched medical advice, which empowers you to make good decisions about your future and your future health.

I'm not advising you to avoid doctors at all costs: far from it. Establishing a good therapeutic relationship with a GP or gynaecologist whom you respect and trust is probably the first thing you should do. It is certainly something I would advise you to take the time to develop now, just as you would develop a relationship with a potential life-partner, research a new job opportunity or find a new neighbourhood to live in. Your doctor or healer can become a real friend and support for life. But most of the issues that may arise for you in your menopause are matters for your own decision-making. In researching this book, I spoke to many, many women, from all over the world, and asked them to share their experiences of menopause. These women were mostly strangers, responding to emails that I initially circulated to friends and colleagues seeking their experiences and words of advice; these were passed on to other post- and peri-menopausal women who were willing to contribute to the book. The response has been enormously generous. These women's words have been quoted extensively throughout the chapters, and I hope that you find as much value and inspiration in their wisdom and experience as I did.

In this book, I want to give you as much medical and scientific information as possible so that you'll feel empowered and informed to take real control of your menopausal life. But I also want to show you how, with proper scientific examination of the research done on the menopause and ageing in women, we can manage the unpleasant symptoms in a natural, drug-free way. With good, scientifically proven information, you can learn to manage the symptoms of menopause, and develop a health strategy in your mid-life that stays with you for the future. Properly informed, we can use this time of menopause fruitfully – to protect our bones, to protect ourselves against cancer and heart disease, and to protect our most important body part of all: our minds.

1

What really happens to my body during menopause?

Last week I bumped into my friend Olivia. She looked stunning. The last time I'd seen Olivia was at a party, four years previously. She was overweight, and looked uncomfortable and sad. She was obviously unhappy in her body; she wanted to look nice but was unable to face wearing an evening dress. While younger, slimmer women danced around the room she sat miserably, watching her husband flit about and chat, ever popular. When I talked to her I found her just her usual self: sweet, intelligent, interested in life, fun and stimulating to talk to. But she looked 'not-herself'. Her hair was greying and made her appear elderly. She was lumpy-looking in a long-sleeved top that did nothing for her. She seemed uncomfortable, lonely and unhappy. She was 44 years old at the time and looked as though she felt all of 60.

So, when I came across her last week, looking slim, trim, lively and full of energy, I was absolutely thrilled. We chatted happily for about half an hour and I couldn't stop complimenting her. She responded by laughing, but we didn't dwell on her transformation. There was so much more to talk about: her new job, developments at home, her daughter's career success. Olivia was a different person, and despite being four years older than when I'd last met her, she seemed ten years younger.

'You look amazing,' I kept saying, and she eventually stopped dismissing my compliments and told me about the dance classes she was going to three times a week, and which were partly the reason for her weight loss. 'I put on a lot of weight, in my mid-forties,' she reminded me. Her weight had just ballooned and she'd felt she had absolutely no control over the way her body was growing. Her breasts had grown by two cup sizes and she had resorted to buying bras online. She'd gone up three dress sizes. She was often breathless and unable to exercise, and didn't seem able to do anything to improve matters. Her job had run into a crisis and she and her husband had stopped having sex.

What was terrifying her most, at that time, was what lay ahead. 'If I'm this unfit at the age of 44,' Olivia had asked herself, 'how on earth am I going to cope at 60?' She felt exhausted all the time, hot and bothered, depressed, and unable to enjoy life. Now 48, Olivia is slim and energetic again. 'What changed?' I asked her. She shrugged. 'I was going through the menopause. Between the years of 44 and 48 it was as if I had been given a different body. I just wasn't myself and I didn't know how to feel like myself. I'd been given the body of a fat old lady and expected to deal with it! And so I had to try to get to know myself again, and that took a bit of thought and effort. But then, after the hot flushes and the few years around that were over, I did become able to cope with life again. My appetite for large fatty meals and chocolate went away. I became quite satisfied with small meals, and now I'm only really interested in healthy food. I exercise, sleep better and have much more energy. I feel as though I'm in control of my body again. It sprouted out in all directions for a number of years, it sweated and ached and felt as though it belonged to someone else, and then it just settled down again and I got back to being me!'

We laughed and thought about this. I told Olivia about this book, on which I was working at the time, and asked her for her thoughts: something wise that she'd love to share with other women. 'Menopause', Olivia said, 'is like puberty for adults. You're happily going along enjoying adult life, just the way kids are enjoying childhood. Then, all of a sudden, your body changes overnight. Nothing looks the same. You're a different shape, you smell different, feel different, your emotions are all over the place. You don't know yourself. You try to confide in people to get help and they either laugh at you or suggest tranquillizers! But then, after a few years, it's suddenly all over. You feel quite normal again, and what's most important, you feel you are yourself. Only this time, you're more mature, wiser and much happier than you've ever been. You've got a different body from the one you had in your thirties, but it's no longer out of control. It's your body and you can enjoy and look after it. You know how to do this, and it's going to be fine. It's just ageing. And it's kind of fun.'

Why a drug-free menopause?

Before I set out to write this book, I sent a brief questionnaire around to every menopausal and post-menopausal woman I know, asking them to describe their experiences and to offer any advice they thought might help those who would read the book, and to pass this request on to others. Some of the responses appear throughout the book, and I hope you'll enjoy reading them as much as I did! But I began to ask myself, as I documented their words, just how much of our anxiety and discomfort around the menopause is entirely natural to women, and how much is created by a variety of industries. From pharmaceuticals to musicals, menopause has become a force in modern culture. In fact, during the last decades of the twentieth century, the menopause became a massive multinational medical industry.

Hormone replacement therapy (HRT) was developed in the 1920s and 1930s as a treatment for symptoms of menopause, using a product derived from the urine of a pregnant mare. Plenty of concerns were expressed back then, in the medical literature, about the possibility of future undesired effects on women who were given artificial hormones. However, the American Drug Manufacturers Association lobbied massively to dispel these concerns, and so oestrogen products were approved by the Food and Drug Administration (FDA) in 1941 for the direct symptoms of menopause: hot flushes and night sweats, vaginal dryness and atrophy (shrinking). In the following decades, oestrogen (either alone or combined with progesterone) gained massive approval among doctors as a complete antidote to many of the illnesses and afflictions of ageing, and was even prescribed as a preventative remedy for osteoporosis, heart disease and Alzheimer's.

It had become clear by the 1970s that taking oestrogen led to an increased risk of cancer of the uterus and ovaries, but manufacturers were then quick to switch their recommendation to products that contained both oestrogen and progesterone, claiming that progesterone would 'oppose' the carcinogenic effects of oestrogen.

In 1991, the US National Institute of Health launched the Women's Health Initiative, which aimed to investigate some of the major health problems of older women who were being treated with HRT. The WHI launched a series of trials, comparing women on HRT to those on placebo. The trials found that women who were treated with oestrogen plus progesterone had an increased risk of heart attack, stroke, blood clots and breast cancer. This finding was so unarguable that the trials had to be stopped, and HRT use declined massively all around the world.

We are now in a twilight period as regards hormones in female medicine. The Million Women Study, a study involving women over the age of 50 in the UK, has also found irrefutable links between hormone replacement therapies and breast cancers. Women need to find other ways of tolerating the symptoms of womanhood, which do not kill us or cause us harm.

Last year I had the very good fortune to spend time with the Wampanoag tribe of American Indians in Massachusetts. In their Visitors' Centre is a wall on which is displayed photographs of their leaders, over the decades. For the Wampanoag, seniority is a guarantee of political leadership, without the need for campaigning and election. So, if you're over 60, you automatically become a tribal elder and get to be involved in social policy decisions, the same as in any government. Except, you are awarded your leadership role on the basis of an understanding that your age is a skill in itself. It is an asset. It is a guarantee of wisdom.

The best thing, for me, about these photographs was the fact that most of them are of women. Women outlive men, no matter where we live in the world; and lifestyle would appear not to be an issue – the Wampanoag, for example, are teetotal, and work on the land, not in factories or cities. Among the Wampanoag Indians, the vast majority of tribal elders are women. Contrast this to any European, Australian, or white-American government, regardless of the uptake of HRT!

'Western' society does not reward ageing. It associates the older woman with ridicule, uselessness and emotional instability. Even a fun stage show like *Menopause – The Musical* takes its comedy from the situation of a middle-aged woman trying not to show her age. As menopausal women, we are so used to being made fun of, to the idea of forgetfulness being the point of comedy, to the shamefulness of the uncontrollable hot flush, that we can tend to forget that we are anything *other* than a menopausal woman.

For many women, their menopause becomes their every day. It becomes their work, their relationship, their friendships, their holidays, their hobby. It overtakes their life. For others, menopause is just a convenient jargon-word for the period in a woman's life when her fertility cycles end.

What do we mean by menopause?

So if menopause is not just an industry, what exactly *do* we mean when we talk about menopause? And how come it causes so much misery? Menopause means, literally, the last period: 'meno' from 'menses', or menstrual period, and 'pause' meaning the last one. However, generally when we talk about menopause we mean the five to ten years around which the last period happens, which for most women is around 50. Realistically, this means anywhere between 40 and 60, although the average age of menopause is 51. Bear in mind, though, that the average woman doesn't exist!

But even if you were the average woman, how would you know that it's your last period, until you haven't had another? Doctors define the 'last period' or menopause as the period you had at least a year before you never had another period again. So, if you have a period at 45, and then 11 months later have another period at the age of 46, technically you haven't actually had your 'menopause'. Many women splutter along like this for several years in their late forties, until they have their final period at (again, on average!) the age of 50. So when you haven't had a period for over two years, you can say for sure that you are definitely infertile and are most certainly post-menopausal.

The majority of women experience 'menopausal symptoms' long before the last period: 80 per cent of women find that they have hot flushes, vaginal dryness and weight gain by their mid-forties. These are generally the first symptoms that alert you to the approach of the menopause: that is, the last period. And 60 per cent of women have their last period within six months of these symptoms being noticed.

Menopause sneaked up on me. I thought the hot flushes and night sweats were to do with drinking too much red wine . . . Well, maybe they were . . . Because I continued having periods until I was about 56 I didn't think the change had actually started. I was, it must be said, loath to let go of my menstrual cycle – I hung on to it for grim death, way past its use-by date – scared I would shrivel up and lose all interest in sex.

I was tied in to a lunar/menstrual pattern I didn't think I'd be able to function without. How, for example, would I know when to clean the house, without my monthly pre-menstrual cleaning madness? How would I explain why I was so awful to everyone without the 'Mittelschmerz' get-out-of-gaol card?

I was working in the show *Menopause – The Musical* when I finally realized everything I was singing and dancing about every night was actually happening to *me*. Well, duhhhh . . .

Lack of confidence: that was the worst thing about it. I actually didn't feel that different physically, or even mentally. I just suddenly realized that my periods stopped when I was 45, and for me that meant that I was going to become old. That scared me and I just lost all my confidence: every little ache and pain became grossly exaggerated! I was terrified of suddenly becoming old.

I panicked if I woke up early thinking I was suffering from depression, I panicked if I didn't get to the gym in case my bones were weakening, I panicked if I gained a few pounds in weight . . . it took me a couple of years to realize that I was just doing fine, and that really, nothing had happened to me apart from the fact that my last period was ages ago. I kind of wish that there wasn't a word for it – menopause – because if we didn't have a word for it, we wouldn't even know it was happening.

Fear of menopause, like fear of most things, was much worse than the actual thing itself.

The 'last period' and loss of oestrogen

Why should the 'last period' be associated with such turmoil? The truth is that medicine isn't very helpful about putting a label on this period of emotional, physical and spiritual turmoil, which involves the end of fertility, the beginning of ageing and the development of massive changes in a woman's physical well-being, such as rapid weight gain, increased cancer risk, hot flushes, leg cramps and loss of libido. But the general assumption has been that changing levels of female fertility hormones, associated with 'ovarian failure' or ageing of the ovaries, has widespread effects on body and mind. Why this should be so, we still don't know. But because menopausal women *felt* better when they were given oestrogen replacement in those early days, it has made sense to medicine that the loss of oestrogen after menopause must have caused all the problems in the first place.

Why is oestrogen so important?

Oestrogen is a hormone, or chemical messenger. All the cells of the body work by receiving chemical messages from other cells: one cell, such as an ovarian cell, secretes an oestrogen 'message' which through the bloodstream reaches other cells of the body that have 'receptors' (areas of the cell wall that understand the message, and know what to do with it). So an oestrogen molecule is actually a message released by an ovarian cell, which can be received by, say, a vaginal cell, which knows to secrete mucus in response to the message, resulting in a moist vaginal environment, conducive to sexuality and fertility.

These are the obvious effects, that we can feel and see, of the oestrogen hormonal cell messages. But oestrogen also has receptors in cells all over the body, as we'll discuss later, and therefore the widespread symptoms of menopause have all been linked to reduction of circulating oestrogens in the bloodstream, after the menstrual cycle ends.

The 'change' – goodbye to all that

For many women, menopause is an opportunity to say goodbye to childbearing, to child-rearing, or perhaps to the possibility of motherhood once and for all, and to say hello to oneself. After menopause, you can no longer reproduce. You are a woman alone, standing still after so many years of cycling the seemingly unending whirl of bloating, cramping, counting pills, using condoms, missing periods, giving birth, bleeding, cursing nature. Everything in your body is getting ready to quieten down. Your busy, bustling, fertile body, which engorged and discharged and squirted and swelled with

> ### How will I know if I've had my last period?
>
> You won't know that it *was* your last until a year after it actually happened! But, while you're waiting, there are several medical ways of checking whether or not your body is fertile. An ultrasound scan of the ovaries can check for lack of ripening follicles, signalling the end of ovarian function. A simple blood test can check for follicle stimulating hormone levels, or for oestrogen levels, as ripe monthly follicles in the ovary secrete oestrogens.
>
> If you still have ovarian function, detectable by ultrasound or blood tests, you can assume that you aren't menopausal and therefore are still potentially fertile. This is useful information if you need to make a decision about whether to use contraception, or keep trying for a baby.

its potential to develop new life while you were a fertile woman, is now settling itself down. It is closing off engorged parts, softening your breasts, coming home to rest. Be gentle on yourself. You are entering a magical phase.

Your menopause is the end of your fertility cycle, but it can become the beginning of something else. For many women, leaving fertility behind can be a new opportunity: to change career, to get the house back after years of child-rearing, or to enter a different relationship phase. Change in your body can be a very good thing. You can use the change to think about what you really want from life, and let your changing mind and body lead you there.

> In Elizabeth Gilbert's memoir *Eat, Pray, Love* the author describes a Buddhist parable about the relationship between the acorn and the oak. She compares herself as a young girl to an acorn, ripe and nubile but also vulnerable and seed-like; then she compares herself as an older woman to an oak tree, hard, strong and solid – but at the same time linked to the acorn, as one has grown into the other.
>
> And so there is a connection between the acorn that she once was, and the oak tree that she will become, the oak tree leading, pulling the acorn behind her. It's easy to forget that you *are* still the same person that you were as a little girl, a teenager, a young woman; you will one day be a much older woman than you are now, and you

will be that same person too. But you *feel* very different when you're middle-aged from how you felt when you were young, and you'll *feel* different again when you're elderly. Because of these strong feelings, and dramatic changes to the world in which we live, it can be easy to forget that there is a very strong connection between all those different women.

Take some time now to think, with love, about the young, vulnerable woman you are leaving behind you, still pulling her with you but at the same time looking fondly back at her as she trails behind you. Think proudly about the woman you have grown into now, looking forward with trepidation and confidence. Finally, think confidently about the even stronger, more powerful woman you are yet to become.

2

All about oestrogen

We are all different. You know yourself better than doctors or other women. You can seek advice, and then take decisions on your own at the end.

Hormones and the menopause

In the healthy female body, there's a relationship between the pituitary and hypothalamus, in the brain, and the ovaries, called the pituitary hypothalamic ovarian axis. This means that the brain organizes your fertility cycle, from your very first period right through all your cycles, every month during your fertile life. The ovaries, situated in the lower part of the abdomen, secrete the fertility hormones oestrogen and progesterone. Levels of these hormones in the bloodstream are constantly monitored by the pituitary gland and hypothalamus in the brain, so that the brain knows what the fertile body is doing: a system that in medicine we call *feedback*.

The brain produces a hormone that stimulates the ovaries to produce follicles, or ripen eggs, called follicle stimulating hormone (FSH). The ripening follicles then produce oestrogen, the female 'feel-good' hormone. Once the follicles have produced sufficient oestrogen in the blood, the brain notices this oestrogen level and responds by producing another hormone, luteinizing hormone, which causes the follicle to burst and die. The ripe follicle ruptures, and as a result of this, the womb sheds its lining as a menstrual period. Every month – or thereabouts.

The brain now knows that you have not been fertilized during this cycle, and so it needs to start to stimulate the ovaries again. It immediately begins a new fertility cycle, stimulating the follicles just enough to ripen, getting feedback all the time from the oestrogens and progesterones that are being produced by the ovaries.

The menopause is the total end of the menstrual cycle, the cycle in which follicles are ripened every month, producing oestrogen to line the uterus in preparation for pregnancy.

'Peri-menopausal' and 'post-menopausal' explained

Doctors regard a woman as peri-menopausal during the last two years of her menstrual cycle, and post-menopausal when she had her last period two years ago. This sounds a bit vague, but the reason for the two-year idea is that it is easy for doctors to make a note of your last period, and then calculate your risk of menopausal-related symptoms based on that. Doctors like numbers, calendar dates and measurements in general! But if you are still getting some periods every now and then, or if you had a period, say, nine months ago, you are in what doctors call the peri-menopause. By this they mean that your fertility is certainly diminished, and that you will probably have your last period within the next two years, if you haven't already had it. If your last period was over two years ago, you are definitely menopausal, and you will not become pregnant again.

Post-menopausal is a term that doctors find useful as it defines fertility: the ovaries have ceased to function. Any bleeding from the womb or vagina after the ovaries have ceased to function is called 'post-menopausal bleeding', and it is always abnormal. Therefore, knowing that you've definitely had your last period is useful to you as any bleeding after that will need to be investigated.

Irregular periods – the first sign of menopause?

Towards mid-life, the ovaries produce fewer follicles. So, what you might notice at first is that your periods become more frequent. This is because your brain is responding to the shortage of follicles, and to the realization that your fertility opportunities may be in jeopardy. The brain stimulates a new follicle when an old one has just burst and dropped its egg into the womb. But if the stimulus from the ovary isn't strong enough, in middle life, for the brain to feel satisfied that the follicle is ripe enough, it quickly responds by stimulating the ripening of another follicle from the ovary. And another, and another. For many women this is a difficult time, when one period seems almost to run into the next, and you might feel as though you are trapped in a cycle of bloating, bleeding, bloating, bleeding, with absolutely no respite from your hormones.

Some women may bleed very heavily around this time as well. Your womb is responding to the direction it receives from your brain, which is to clear out the old lining as efficiently as possible, because it's time for a new follicle to be ripened. However, many of these follicles are too weak to become fertile in the first place, and so the feedback to the brain is not as strong as you might have had during your fertile years. Your womb may bleed heavily, while at the same time your body is stimulating itself to produce another follicle, which causes even heavier bleeding next time. Some women develop fibroid swellings in the womb around this time, as the womb struggles to do its work. If your bleeding is becoming a problem to you in terms of pain, weakness or fainting, or if it is impossible to conduct daily life or go to work, please see your gynaecologist and have an examination of the womb, ovaries and vagina.

Contraception – should I still be using it?

My periods are very infrequent; I had my last one over a year ago, but I'm only in my mid-forties. Should I still be using contraception?

There is no simple answer to this question! A long time since your last period *might* mean that you're finished with your ovarian function, but there are other, reversible causes for your periods to stop too: poor diet, stress, thyroid disease, pituitary disease. Therefore, if your periods have stopped unexpectedly you should consult with your doctor; lack of periods doesn't necessarily mean that you are completely infertile. You need to be sure about the cause before stopping all contraception.

After the menopause, the body secretes very low levels of follicle stimulating hormone and luteinizing hormone; a simple blood test can detect this, which helps to discover whether you have definitely finished with your fertility cycle. But the blood test alone is not enough. As a rule of thumb, doctors say that women above the age of 50 who have had no period for over 12 months, and who have hot flushes, can stop using contraception. If it isn't a full year since your last period, a simple foam or spermicide contraceptive would do.

A trans-vaginal ultrasound can detect whether or not you still have any follicles on your ovaries, but this is an invasive procedure that is somewhat uncomfortable, so don't feel that you need to have this test done, if a simple blood test is available. The trans-vaginal ultrasound can be very useful if you are trying for a baby during this time. Problematic periods may be another reason why your doctor would want to examine your ovaries, womb and internal organs in this way, so if you are experiencing irregular or abnormal bleeding, or pain, or have any concern about the symptoms of your menopause, this examination can help your doctor to investigate for cancer of the womb, cervix and ovaries.

During peri-menopause, or below the age of 50, there is still a risk that your ovary could ripen another egg, and women do become pregnant in their late forties, when they least expect it. So please consult with your doctor before you decide that you are definitely finished with your family. Progesterone-only contraceptive pills, the Mirena coil, and progesterone implants under the skin of your arm, are all currently recommended for use around menopause. Oestrogen-containing pills are generally not prescribed for women over 45 as they are associated with a higher risk of clots and cancers.

Condoms, caps and diaphragms are all useful contraceptives in your forties and fifties, and don't require you to take any artificial hormones into your body. A vasectomy is also a safe, drug-free way of avoiding pregnancy.

Heavy bleeding – when should I be concerned?

How much heavy bleeding around the time of peri-menopause is too heavy? When should I be concerned?

Roughly, you should never pass clots bigger than a two-pound/euro coin. If you are using more than one pack of tampons or towels in any one period, this is probably too heavy. You should never have pain that interferes with your ability to work or live day to day. In either case, consult your gynaecologist.

A simple ultrasound scan shows any fibroids, benign growths of the lining of the womb, that can cause problematic bleeding. A trans-vaginal ultrasound scan can be used to examine the ovaries fully and screen for ovarian cancer. A vaginal examination enables the gynaecologist to check your internal pelvic organs and detect any abnormality in their size or shape, or if there are fibroids or lumps. She will be able to examine the ovaries, to look for any abnormality in size, or if there is tenderness there. She can also answer any of your concerns that you might be having about menopause, your periods, or any bleeding problems you've had. She can check your vagina and take samples of fluids to check for sexually transmitted diseases (STDs) or other causes of discharge, odour, bleeding or pain.

You should also ensure that you have an up-to-date smear test. A smear-taker should inspect the visual appearance of your internal vagina and cervix as she passes the speculum. Polyps or any other cervical cause of bleeding can usually be seen this way.

Unpicking the myths

Between 60 and 80 per cent of women complain of some sort of physical symptom during menopause. Most of these symptoms are temporary, and few are of 'significance', in that they are not associated with disease. The symptoms are uncomfortable, often humiliating, yet much of this is because of the way menopause does not fit with the busy, modern, highly stressed female life, with its demands on our energy, our beauty, our labour and our attention to others.

In many ways, the reality of female life is shrouded behind the 'ideal' image of womanhood: a woman who runs, swims and plays tennis during her period, smells fragrant, and whose body is pimple-free, toned, and with perfectly symmetrical genitalia that have been airbrushed for a garage calendar. Despite the giant multinational industry that menopause and hormone replacement has become, women's bodies are still a mystery to many, even to their owners. And, in many ways, the attempt by the pharmaceutical industries to mask the symptoms of menopause, to cover up the effects of ageing, to make women 'forever feminine', have simply perpetuated the unspoken taboo surrounding the ageing woman.

We cannot fully be prepared for the effect that menopause will have on our bodies, as every woman's experience will be different. However, in contrast to the menarche, or first period, our last period at least comes during a time when we are much more in control of our lives.

Actually, for me it was a blessing. I went through menopause without noticing; I think my body decided that it didn't need one more thing to tax itself. My mother, on the other hand, had hot flushes until she was in her eighties.

Oestrogen and the menopause

So why does the menopause make women feel so awful? The answer is connected to the reduction in oestrogen. It's important to remember that oestrogen doesn't disappear after menopause – it still circulates in the body, albeit at much lower levels. This post-menopausal oestrogen comes from the adrenal glands, beside the kidneys, and by about six months after the last period levels are lower than 30 international units (IU) per ml.

Oestrogen and progesterone have a relationship with all the tissues and cells with the body, not just with the womb and follicles. We already know that they operate very closely with the brain, and doctors now believe that oestrogen in particular has a strong relationship with the breasts, skin, bones, as well as the heart and blood vessels, and of course, the lining tissues of the vagina and reproductive passage. This means that the reduction in circulating oestrogens will affect all the tissues in your body. It might be tempting to regard these changes as 'ageing', but really, it is simply a maturation of your body as your fertile period ceases, and your new, independent and self-oriented period begins.

Oestrogen and the heart

Many doctors feel that oestrogen must have a protective effect on the blood vessels and cardiovascular system, as women who are post-menopausal have a much higher risk of heart disease. Some doctors have assumed that when oestrogen levels become low, the blood vessels in the skin dilate or expand, which is what causes hot flushes. This may or may not be the case, but it is true that after middle age your risk of heart or blood pressure problems, palpitations and swollen feet increases. So, you need to take very good care of your heart and vessels from now on (see Chapters 6 and 10).

Oestrogen and the reproductive organs

You may notice that your vagina seems dryer, or that you find sex uncomfortable. If you have had children and a vaginal delivery, your womb, or cervix, may seem lower, or 'in the way'. You may find that you get more urinary tract infections (UTI), cystitis, or that you feel burning or discomfort after sex, or when you pass urine. Or that your urine smells foul. All these symptoms are thought to be because of the reduction of circulating oestrogens, which have a relationship with your vagina, bladder and internal organs of reproduction. Oestrogen, during fertile life, has a moisturizing effect on these cells (see Chapter 3).

Oestrogen and the bones

Oestrogen seems to have a positive effect on your bones, which means that women after menopause are more likely to develop osteoporosis, osteopenia, or thinning and demineralization of the bones, than earlier in life. Loss of your periods means that you now must take your bone health seriously, and develop an exercise and bone health strategy for life (see Chapter 5).

Oestrogen and body fluids

During the menstrual cycle, bloating can be troublesome to many women. Bloating is your body's natural tendency to retain water and salt just before your period; it is a side-effect of the hormones that your brain is producing to stimulate your ovaries and womb. These menstrual hormones affect the kidneys, liver and internal organs of the abdomen as well as the ovaries and womb, and so you naturally feel puffy and bloated before and during a period.

Oestrogen and the brain

We know from our discussion about the menstrual cycle that oestrogen stimulates the brain. But, while your brain is sensitive to oestrogen, it is not an oestrogen sponge! There are many other factors around the time of menopause that have an effect on mood: stress, worry, overwork, being rushed or pressured, poor nutrition, too much coffee and tea, not drinking enough water, too much alcohol . . .

Evening primrose oil

For many women just before the menopause, bloating becomes extreme. It can feel very uncomfortable. Drinking plenty of water helps, as does eating less salt and drinking less alcohol and drinks containing caffeine, as these all contribute to water retention.

Evening primrose oil is a natural herbal remedy which in high doses has been found in trials to relieve to some extent bloating in the peri-menopause, and it is safe to take throughout life. It is also thought to have a positive effect on bone health, and in arthritis, where it is recommended in doses of up to 2,500 mg per day. As many of the capsules come in 300 mg doses, you would need to take quite a few of these.

Cutting back on stress, work-overload and worry will make a huge difference, and later in the book we'll talk about effective strategies for mindfulness and developing neurological activity during menopause. Studies have shown that during the time of menopause many women become more productive, more imaginative, and more creative than ever before, as some of the troublesome worries, such as child-rearing or unfulfilling employment, can be removed, and as they gain the maturity and self-esteem to take on new challenges and develop more power.

My experience isn't the usual, but from others I wonder about the balance between the psychological and physical and how to determine how to deal with both. There seems to be some connection between moving out of your fertile years and becoming invisible in your world – a hard pill to swallow for some, but a welcome relief for others.

3

How do I cope with hot flushes?

If a menopausal woman has pain or makes trouble, pound her hard on the jaw.

(Egyptian medical text dated 2000 BC)

My doctor was not even remotely interested in helping me with any symptom control, I had to research this myself and take appropriate supplements, using trial and error. Soya drinks were a comfort for me as well as exercise, mainly swimming.

An unbearable symptom?

So there you are, sitting at an important meeting. It might be at work. It might be a parent–teacher meeting. It might be a job interview, a date, a session with a client, a difficult conversation with your boss, an important conversation with your friend: it matters not. The point is that you've got to make sure that you're making yourself understood, that your communication is effective. Except that your face feels as if someone has just shoved it into an oven. Your entire body is drenched in sweat. It's a blustery winter's day outside, but here in this room you feel as though you're sitting in a sauna. The windows are closed. The room is an inferno! Everybody must be staring at you! It's a menopausal hot flush, you can do nothing about it and EVERYBODY KNOWS.

I've put the last bit in capitals because, let's be honest, that's probably the worst thing about the whole hideous event. The fact that you genuinely believe that you can't hide what's happening to you.

When I was researching this book I asked every menopausal and post-menopausal woman I know, what was the thing that affected her most. The results were quite astonishing. Women who were still in, or approaching the menopause, almost universally complained that the hot flushes were an absolutely unbearable symptom of menopause. This is a typical response:

> The only signs of menopause I ever got were hot flushes. I had to have the windows open all the time, in the car, in the house, even in winter. They were extremely distressing. They were very frequent, at their worst every 30 minutes or so, and extreme – whole upper-body sweats, extreme heat and redness. I tried numerous remedies and came to the conclusion that the only thing that worked was HRT. I took this for five years. I still have the flushes, but they are much reduced.

My heart broke when I read that woman's email. As I pictured her, trapped in her car with the windows down, I could almost feel the despair in her voice. But, it was very interesting what women who are past their menopause told me: women who've finished their menopause don't remember the hot flushes. Well, they recall them if you ask them specifically, but they shrug them off and tell you, 'Well, perhaps I did have one or two but they didn't really affect me.'

Now, how does this add up? I surveyed well over a hundred women still in their menopause: pretty much all of them moaned and groaned about the awful hot flushes. And I surveyed pretty much the same number of women who'd had their menopause, some up to 20 years ago. They could barely remember them.

You may be concluding that post-menopausal women are desperately forgetful, or that they had all been on HRT. But I thought of that too, and I was careful only to talk to women who had never had HRT; most were still working and active in an intellectual environment, contacts of mine or through friends – doctors, writers, mothers, grandmothers, teachers, nurses, and so on.

I became very curious when I started to talk to women who claimed that they couldn't remember any menopausal 'symptoms'. How did you know, I asked all of these women, if you can't even remember the symptoms, that you were in the menopause? This is what one woman, now aged 62, told me.

> Well, my periods stopped, I suppose. But actually, it was about a year or two after they'd stopped before I realized that I wasn't going to have another one! I was very busy at the time, my kids were at university, I was making a huge breakthrough in my career. My husband and I started

travelling a lot and we visited lots of very exciting places. I can't remember having had time to worry about the menopause!

Now, I happen to remember this woman very well when she was 55; she was sitting in a very important meeting, fanning herself like crazy, running to the door and back to get some cool air, feeling hideously embarrassed. But this probably happened so infrequently, compared to all the wonderful things she remembers about that time (her career success, her children's achievements, her wonderful experiences travelling with her husband) that she can't actually remember having been troubled by those flushes. This is not a unique experience. People filter memories and experiences all the time.

But here you still are, thinking that your hot flushes are absolutely unbearable and so you don't want to hear about other women who've conquered theirs. Fair enough. Let's think about *your* hot flushes, and how you can cope with them.

Understanding hot flushes

Being terrified of hot flushes is guaranteed to make sure that they are worse, no matter what age or gender you are. Studies show that women have hot flushes right through life, and long before the periods stop, if we measure day-to-day temperature fluctuations. But, it's only around the menopause that they cause problems.

Most women say that they can't predict when hot flushes begin, nor how long they will last. But once we start to understand why the hot flush is happening, what causes it, how long it lasts, we can start to feel in control. And there are many drug-free methods of reducing the effects and frequency of hot flushes.

Hot flushes occur in up to 40 per cent of regularly menstruating women in their forties. The vast majority, roughly 80 per cent of women, will be finished with them after five years. In over 50 per cent of women the hot flushes last less than one year, in 40 per cent of women less than six months. Sometimes (in about 10 per cent of women), hot flushes can last as long as ten years. But there is no way to predict, in an individual woman, when hot flushes will cease, though they do tend to decrease in frequency over time.

What happens in a hot flush?

Every doctor will tell you that flushes are 'caused' by 'fluctuations in hormonal levels during menopause'. But what they might not tell you is that this is only a theory. How the reduction in oestrogen affects the sweat glands, the sensory nerves in the face, and the general feeling of temperature in the body is actually unknown. However, most gynaecologists say that oestrogen has an effect on the skin, therefore it must affect the sweat glands. It has an effect on the micro-capillaries of the cardiovascular system, therefore it must have a role in dilating and contracting these micro-capillaries during blushing. Again, the exact role has yet to be discovered. And, most gynaecologists also say that oestrogen has an affect on the hypothalamus, the brain centre where the oestrogen/progesterone cycle of periods and fertility is controlled. The hypothalamus controls the body's core temperature. But how, or whether, diminishing levels of oestrogen during menopause cause the body's core temperature to be noticeably elevated is not actually understood.

The truth is that the body temperature does not actually rise to any grand level during a hot flush. You feel hot, but your core temperature remains pretty much the same. The sweat glands feel active, but if you measure moisture on the skin, the amount of sweat you produce during a hot flush does not markedly increase. And, most interestingly, although you genuinely feel, during a hot flush, that your face has become tomato red, it hasn't. Have a look in the mirror. Your skin colour has probably remained the same. Some women experience flushing or blushing across the chest, but generally, unless you have drunk alcohol or taken other substances that may be contributing to the flushing, the face remains the same.

Are hot flushes universal to all women?

On a worldwide scale, menopausal hot flushes are, in fact, not that common. Studies of Japanese, Korean and other Southeast Asian women have found that hot flushes are rarely recorded. Many doctors have theorized that a high intake of soya products, rather than dairy, in Asian diets helps with hot flushes. But we can't actually explain scientifically how plant-based oestrogens affect the cell receptors for oestrogen in the skin. Another puzzling fact is that if you measure the oestrogen levels in women who have hot flushes against those in women who don't, the levels are the same. Therefore, you might extrapolate that the actual oestrogen levels in our own bodies don't appear to be causing the flushes. Yet when the pharmaceutical industry went to research all possible causes of these bothersome symptoms of menopause, they found, to their great advantage, that giving women oestrogen tablets relieved the symptoms. Some of the time.

Nothing lasts

I say 'some of the time', because if you remember the words of the woman who described her five years of hot flush misery, her HRT did relieve her flushes to an extent, in that she now had fewer of them: but it didn't take them away completely. She still had them, long past her menopause. In fact, this is not an unusual occurrence. But I was sobered by this woman's experience of menopause; she's certainly been through it, hasn't she? She's battled with the flushes. She's had the HRT. So what advice would she give to other women now?

I went back to her and asked her this: 'Based on your own experience of managing your own menopause, what "golden" advice would you like to give other women, and why?' This is what she said: 'As Buddhists say, "Nothing lasts".'

I had to smile at this. From a woman who'd had to resort to taking carcinogenic hormones for five years because she couldn't cope without having her car and house windows open constantly, the wisest words of all.

The truth is that a hot flush itself doesn't last – on average, it lasts five seconds. Five seconds from the beginning of the symptom (oh my God, I'm going to have a hot flush!) to the end of the peak of the sensation (OK, it's going away right now).

From my research on post-menopausal women, what I've found out includes the following:

- The average woman has hot flushes for about six months.
- The average woman has between one and five hot flushes per day, for about three months, and then dwindles down to three per week or less.

- And the average woman, when asked, 20 years on, if her hot flushes made a big difference to her life, will tell you that she can't remember them.

The science of hot flushes

Wayne State University School of Medicine in Michigan have been studying hot flushes for 25 years. They have measured women's skin temperature, sweat production, flow of blood to the skin and basal core body temperature, before, during and after hot flushes. They have rigged women up to monitors to collect hot flush data of electrical conductivity in the skin, got them to swallow radioactive pills to measure core body temperature at various different points inside the body, and had them spend the night in a specially constructed sleep laboratory, where all evidence of hot flushes was recorded while they weren't even aware they were having them, during their sleep.

What they have found is that all women have variations of core body temperature during menopausal years. But it should be remembered that we have variations of core body temperature throughout our fertile life, with a peak in temperature being associated with ovulation. For decades women used this method successfully (known as the Billings method after the doctor who first described it) in order to prevent or plan conception. How come these women didn't notice that they 'felt' hot? What was the rectal thermometer every day all about? Surely, if a woman can be so sensitive to changes in her temperature core, so sensitive that she feels the need to take HRT to get rid of this sensation of temperature change, then she would have been just as sensitive to her core temperature during her fertile years, and would never have needed to use contraception because she would have known when she was fertile? I think you might know what the answer is to this.

When Dr Freedman at the Wayne State University School of Medicine measured the core temperature fluctuations of menopausal women, he found that women who complain of hot flushes have a lower 'tolerance' for small increases in the core body temperature than the women who didn't 'have' hot flushes. In other words, if you aren't particularly looking out for fluctuations of temperature, you won't notice them. The women who had hot flushes were those who, when their body naturally varied in core temperature, were the ones who noticed.

Ancient wisdom

Healers in the ancient Ayurvedic tradition have a different way of evaluating symptoms and systems from western medicine, but one feature of health that they always consider is body heat. Certain foods are considered to be heating, and other foods are cooling. Ayurveda suggests that to keep cool you should avoid icy drinks, but instead drink water or freshly blended fruit juices at room temperature.

Rice, bread, milk, butter, melon, cherries, pears, grapes, pineapple, mangoes, cucumber, broccoli, courgettes and asparagus are all considered to be cooling foods. If you have an overheated body temperature, avoid salty, sour and spicy foods: citrus fruits, hot spices, as well as tomatoes, hot peppers, radishes, onions and garlic, and also yoghurt. Cook with cooling spices such as fennel, mint, coriander rather than ginger or mustard.

Making sense of hot flushes

Most women have what's known as a thermoneutral zone of several tenths of a degree centigrade. This means that the body feels pretty OK about its core temperature when it's anywhere between about 36.5 and about 37.5.

What Dr Freedman discovered when he measured the core body temperature of menopausal women with and without hot flushes, was that women with hot flushes had a thermoneutral zone that was 'virtually non-existent'. In other words, the women with hot flushes were really, really aware of their tiny fluctuations in body temperature, whereas women who didn't have hot flushes were having exactly the same fluctuations, it's just that they weren't aware of them.

Freedman's research explains why different women complain differently about the same symptoms, when the exact same body changes happen to every woman throughout the world. It explains why different cultures experience menopause differently. And it explains why, when you're having hot flushes, they are horrendous.

And why, afterwards, when you haven't experienced one for years, you can barely remember them.

Coping with hot flushes

Pay attention to your body and what's happening to it

It's known that if your body is struggling with toxins, this will result in a raise in body temperature. If you hate having hot flushes, consider your body as you load it with toxins such as alcohol, caffeine and maybe tobacco, and think about giving it less work to do.

Consider your liver as it works hard to deal with the huge sugar rush that has been dumped into it every time you eat a carb-heavy food. Refined carbs such as white bread, potatoes, sweets, chocolate, cakes and biscuits all contain high quantities of sugar. This intake of sugar stimulates a surge in insulin, forcing the liver to rapidly metabolize this excess sugar, which is then stored as fat. No wonder you're overheating a bit, if you're enjoying pasta, followed by chocolate cake, with a large glass of wine: your liver is doing overtime. (See Chapter 6 for more on healthy eating.)

The beauty about the body is that many of the things we do naturally and healthily produce heat and sweating, and redden our faces in a way we don't mind at all: dancing to a favourite song, running through an autumn forest, playing tennis with a friend, practising yoga, having a hot, scented bubble bath, being in a sauna in a beautiful day-spa – even having an orgasm. During these experiences, women rarely complain that they can't stand the heat! It's the inappropriateness of the menopausal hot flush that drives us crazy, not the actual body heat.

But why should it? Why shouldn't you be sensitive to your body's core? Sensitivity to the body is a force for good. If your body is heating, listen to it. What have you just eaten, that perhaps may not suit it? What are you wearing that your body doesn't like? Have you been drinking alcohol, and is this really what your body needs at this time in your life? Have you been taking medicines or headache pills, smoking cigarettes, or putting any other unnatural substance into your body that it may now be struggling to excrete?

Keeping a hot flush diary will help you to figure out which environmental factors may be contributing to hot flushes. Take a note of the time of day you have a major flush, the levels of stress on a scale of 1 to 10, what you've just eaten or drunk, and what you were wearing, doing, and so on. You may well begin to notice a pattern.

If you are very troubled by hot flushes, please take some time to think about why these tiny fluctuations in body temperature upset you so much. Then, if you can, actually measure your temperature during a hot flush. You will be astonished to find how little it has actually fluctuated. This is good. It means that you are not actually boiling like a ham in front of all your friends, you are merely being very sensitive to your body's core. Your menopause is a time when you *should* become more sensitive to your own body. You may have spent over 30 years nurturing others: your relationship, your children, your career. Your body is now telling you to nurture yourself. Listen to your core, and as it heats, observe the waves of sensation it is bringing you. Your body is not battling with you, it is asking you to observe it, to listen to it, to feel its changes; it is asking you to honour the changes that it wants to make.

Pay attention to your diet

For many women, changing their diet has been a life-saver in terms of hot flushes. The Royal College of Obstetricians and Gynaecologists suggests that there is some evidence that phyto-oestrogens (most significantly isoflavones found in soybeans, chickpeas and red clover and other legumes) and lignans (oil seeds such as flaxseed, present in cereals, vegetables, legumes and fruits) or isoflavone supplementation may help in some small way with menopausal symptoms. Many women report much improved symptoms by reducing their meat and dairy intake and basing their diet on soya foods, which contain plant-based oestrogens. So, snack on roasted soy nuts, and add tofu to curry, soup or casseroles rather than meat or chicken. Use soy milk on cereal and in tea, switch from dairy to soy cheese, from meat to Quorn, and enjoy miso, tempeh or soy sauce on vegetables instead of salt. Chickpeas and sweet potatoes are also rich in plant oestrogens and can easily be added to all kinds of hot dishes and salads; and eat hummus in sandwiches or on toast rather than butter or mayo.

Some common herbs may have oestrogenic properties, such as nutmeg, oregano, thyme, turmeric and licorice. However, take note if you've had oestrogen-receptive cancer: it isn't known if the oestrogens in plants affect breast or ovarian/uterine tissues in the long term, and so before switching your diet to include much more plant-based oestrogens please discuss this idea with your oncologist.

Herbal remedies

Some studies have found that herbal and non-pharmaceutical medicines help greatly with hot flushes. Of these, black cohosh has had a good deal of success and can reduce or remove hot flushes altogether within about two weeks; however, this remedy should not be taken for more than three months, and as it can cause impaired liver function, you should not take it if you are a heavy drinker, or on any liver enzyme-inducing medicines.

Agnus castus is an ancient remedy for gynaecological conditions that dates back 2,500 years and can be effective for hot flushes. It is available in health-food shops and chemists and is relatively safe in menopause, although it can cross-react with psychiatric drugs, nor should you take it if you have any illness that affects the hormone prolactin.

Read the packaging carefully for any herbal remedy that you decide to try; if in any doubt, consult with your pharmacist or doctor. Although many women report improved symptoms on these botanical products, or Chinese herbal remedies such as ginseng or dong quai, the long-term safety of these medicines has not been measured and therefore they are currently not recommended by licence for the management of menopause.

Mixed 'menopause' products are available that combine (usually) cod liver or fish oil with vitamin E, evening primrose oil, and often one of either black cohosh or agnus castus, green tea extract, vitamin D, calcium and so on, producing a sort of catch-all remedy for the risk factors of menopause. These tablets can be expensive, and the individual dose of each vitamin or fish oil contained in each combined tablet is often not enough to control symptoms, in which case you are better off buying the individual remedies separately. Some women have found that a high dose of vitamin E (1,000 IU) helps with hot flushes, and many studies have found that high-dose evening primrose oil (up to 3,000 mg per day) improves symptoms.

Cooling breath: the ultimate hot flush power solution

Deep 'belly breathing' can bring instant relief to hot flushes. When we take full, deep breaths into our lungs, we allow the body naturally to eliminate heat through the massive volume of water vapour we exhale in every breath. Most of the time we tend to take frequent quick, shallow breaths, only exchanging air very slowly from the top of our lungs. Take some time to breathe deeply, allowing the belly to rise and fall as it is pushed down by the lungs filling with clean, fresh air. Then breathe out as deeply as you can, letting go of as much heat as possible through the lungs.

- Sit or lie down comfortably, letting your hands rest by your side or on your lap. Let the shoulders relax and let go of any tension in the body. Notice your feelings: 'I feel hot', 'I feel in control', 'I feel powerful.'
- Notice your breath. With each breath, breathe deeply through the nostrils into the lungs, from the collar bone through the chest and deep into the back, noticing your belly rise and swell as you fill your lungs with air. With each exhalation, let your belly fall naturally with the air from the deepest part of your lungs, chest, collar bone. Exhale completely before you take the next deep, deep breath, all the time focusing on your belly rising and falling.
- Notice your feelings: 'I feel calm', 'I feel cool', 'I feel alive', 'I feel energized', 'I feel grateful', 'I feel empowered.'
- When you feel it's time to stop, pinch yourself on the wrist. This will anchor the good feelings, and remind you to do this again, next time you are bothered by hot flushes!

Jan's story

Jan was struggling with headaches and hot flushes, desperate to find a solution as the symptoms were really interrupting her enjoyment of life. But her mother had died of breast cancer and so HRT was out of the question. Her doctor had no suggestions to help with the hot flushes.

Jan's sister had given up dairy products several years previously, due to dietary problems, and she had never been bothered with menopausal symptoms. Jan asked her sister whether she thought that the diet she'd been on had helped with menopause. Her sister wasn't sure if it was the diet, but she had definitely had an easier time in menopause than Jan! So Jan did some research and discovered that women in China and Japan don't suffer particularly severe effects from the menopause and this is attributed to the fact that they don't eat dairy products. She was amazed to discover that incidents of breast cancer are also very low in these countries.

Jan learned about how during the menopause oestrogen levels are depleted, and this is what is thought to cause a lot of menopausal problems. Soy mimics oestrogen and therefore possibly explains why Chinese women sail through the menopause. Jan didn't cut out dairy completely, but she now takes two to three servings of soya products every day. She quickly realized that soya yogurts taste just the same as dairy ones, and that you can buy frozen soya beans that taste the same as peas. Since changing her diet Jan's headaches have definitely eased off. She is slimmer than she was, she's full of energy and looks years younger than her age.

4

Low mood, depression and your emotional well-being

His wife has a lot of different menopausal symptoms, but only a few really irritate him. Her hot flashes, her vertigo, her palpitations – that's her problem. What really bothers him is her nervousness, her irritability, and her excessive anxiety, often expressed by endless 'book-shuffling, chain-smoking, reading-lamp' insomnia! ... [Menrium] takes care of the vasomotor symptoms as well as the emotional symptoms. That means the symptoms that bother his wife the most. And the symptoms that irritate him the most. So, to help them both get through menopause, remember Menrium.

(1960s advert for Hoffmann La Roche's hormone replacement therapy drug, Menrium)

I actually didn't notice a difference when I had my menopause, because my life was very stressful at that time, and I think it took me months to realize that I was no longer having periods!

The first thing I noticed was the tiredness. I didn't realize I had entered the menopause but my energy levels had dropped dramatically. It made me feel really, really depressed.

Menopause and negative feelings

About 40 per cent of women around menopause complain of emotional problems, like weepiness, loss of confidence, mood swings, sadness, or even suicidal feelings. Therefore it has been assumed that menopause is a risk factor for, or is associated with, low mood. But *clinical depression* is no more common during the menopause than at any other time in a woman's life, and any depression during menopause is no different from depression she may be at risk of at any other period of life. The problem with trying to find a reason for all the emotional problems that can arise during the menopause, is that it is difficult to research this area, which is multi-factorial. A risk factor isn't the same thing as a cause. An association isn't the same as causation. Grey hair, for example, is associated with old age. So is high blood pressure. But nobody believes for a moment that grey hair causes your blood pressure to go up! It's just that both are associated with ageing, and they tend to happen around the same time.

Just because you are beginning to change the way you feel about work, love, confidence, friends, solitude, tiredness, staying up late, food, sex, and other aspects of your day-to-day life, this doesn't necessarily mean that something in your body has caused this change. Nor does it mean that these changes are necessarily a bad thing. However, it is true that the bodily and the psychological changes that happen during and after the menopause affect the way you feel about many things.

Many women assume that their negative feelings are because of the menopause. While menopause is certainly associated with reduced sex drive, because of a reduction in circulating oestrogens, and may be associated with disturbed sleep, there is no real physical reason to feel intensely sad, or experience a total loss of energy, or exhaustion, or a lack of confidence, simply because you are no longer having periods. If anything, a simple cessation of the menstrual cycle should be no more emotionally disturbing than childhood, which contained no menstrual cycle whatsoever.

However, we do know from women's experiences that menopause, or climacteric, is a time of intense change.

Climacteric means 'the critical period'. In this critical period, you are entering new territory. You are likely to change the way you work, love, relate to friends, exercise, holiday, eat, drink – and if you don't, your body will struggle with your inability to adapt in order to become the woman of the future that you are destined to be.

Ageing is inevitable, and it is, of course, predictable. What is entirely unpredictable is the way you *feel* about ageing. Does a change in your physical weight cause you distress? For some women it is devastating. Should it cause distress? How much distress? Does an unaccustomed lack of energy for late nights, parties and socializing mean that you have become a negative old frump, whom no one will ever love again? Or does it mean that you have begun to realize that you can do your own thing – you are in charge of your own destiny, and you don't have to put other people first from now on? If you want to retire for an early night with a good book, that is indeed a far better way to spend your time than exhausting yourself with enforced politeness and indifferent company.

If your job has suddenly become boring and meaningless, is it your fault that you are stuck beneath the glass ceiling, that you may be too 'womanly' in a man's world? Or is your job indeed boring and meaningless and would searching for work that inspires you and excites you, regardless of status or income, be something you would consider? These are some of the big questions that women need to ask themselves, before running to the psychiatrist with a giant portion of self-blame for the way we are feeling in the mid-life years.

If your doctor cannot help you to cheer up, you may be tempted to believe that it is your own fault, and thereby it is easy to create a cycle of misery, humiliation and despair. It is well worth your while to take some time during the climacteric, the 'critical period', to take stock of oneself, to slow down, to nurture the spirit and the soul.

Unexpressed anger and stress

Anger, of course, is not a 'feminine' quality. Yet, in a lifetime in which we suffer a childhood interrupted by the explosion of acne, bleeding and cramps that herald our reproductive life, followed by 30 years of menstrual bloating, pain and childbirth, we are then rewarded at the end of this duty to the species with a climacteric storm that bloats our bodies with unwanted fat, curses our joints, slows our muscles, wrinkles our faces, dries up our vaginas and from the point of view of other, younger women and of men, parks us permanently into the unwanted basket of asexual old crones. Angry now? I bet you are! Women aren't expected to feel anger, though, and therefore many of us don't expect to feel it. During the menopausal years we may well become, as more mature adults, aware of perfectly good reasons to feel angry, and yet not know how to actually express this anger efficiently and effectively, as we are so unused to expressing it at all.

Women who have acted as the family 'pacifier' or the office 'listener' may be particularly unable to express anger. We have created a role for ourselves that is to be calm and gentle at all times: a state of being that is physically as well as emotionally unsustainable (unless you have had a lobotomy).

I don't know how I would have coped with menopause, if I hadn't taken up boxing! I was an abused woman and so I learned to kick-box and fight karate during my thirties; it was a confidence-building exercise really but it's kept me sane all these years. I'm 59 now and I go to the boxing gym and teach a boxercise class twice a week. Everything aches, and I often wonder what I'm doing to my body as I grow older! But I had a choice – I could either lie down and die with depression or I could get up and fight. Hitting that punch-bag is what makes my life work for me now. I'm slim and very fit, and very, very strong. Women are full of unexpressed anger, aren't they?

There is nothing wrong with expressing anger. The trick is to know how to express it efficiently, at the right target and in the right sort of way. Anger at the world in general becomes painfully difficult to express if one is stuck at traffic lights, late for an important meeting. Smashed plates will have you spending much valuable time and money in homeware stores rebuying crockery. Acknowledging anger is an important step to actually allowing yourself to feel it. What you do about it, physically and psychologically, and the way in which you choose to express it, is your own adventure.

It's important, therefore, to be very aware of your body as it changes and to become sensitive to what sort of physical *feelings* are quite reasonable and justifiable and deserve physical and emotional expression, and what sort of emotional *reactions* are destructive and will lead to intolerable depression and despair.

I never felt that menopause was a problem for me at all, as I have been doing Traditional Chinese medicine throughout for 15 years. I have no hot flashes, although my family says I have mood swings!

Loss of energy and exhaustion

Menopause can be a time of heightened creativity, when women feel powerful, energized and rejuvenated; they may take on new and exciting projects and interests. This transformation may be quite sudden, as women find themselves freed both from the monthly cycle and very often from childcare as well. But it's also common to notice a gradual decline in energy. Starting a new business in your fifties, for example, may have to be balanced by getting to bed earlier. A work promotion may cause huge difficulty in preventing weight gain, if it means that you will be eating on the hoof.

Many women report a dramatic loss of energy, with feelings of deep exhaustion that lead them to traipse back and forth to their doctor, who takes blood sample after blood sample, without finding any overt physical cause for the tiredness. One of the hardest things for any of us to accept is that after middle age we do need to prioritize rest and peacefulness, and cultivate a gentler pace.

The important thing is to be aware of your changing body and adapt to it. Yes, you need to prioritize sleep and rest, exercise and fresh air from now on. Yes, you need to consider your food intake and your diet much more seriously. Yes, you need to be organized in your personal life so as to make sure you aren't running yourself into the ground by juggling too many balls in the air. And yes, you need to know when your mind and your body are telling you to stop. When to take breaks. When to rest without experiencing guilt, or feeling like a failure.

Combating toxic stress

The physical body, which we may have battered for decades with work, sport, junk food, perhaps cigarettes and alcohol, emotional stress, tension and environmental toxins, does not heal itself as rapidly after menopause as it used to. We can perhaps accept the physical effects of ageing on the skeleton, and make adaptations to that. The spiritual body – the mind – is the more important place to acknowledge, as it may take longer to alert us to its struggle to survive. Less alcohol, fewer carbs, healthy meals in the middle of the day rather than late-night vitamin-free snacks, all make an immediate difference to levels of stress, your mood and how well you sleep.

Taking a rest in the afternoons, for example, is a sensible way of ensuring that you'll have energy to do what you plan to in the evening, or for some work you might want to do in the quiet of the night, when others are out or in bed. It doesn't mean that you've lost your marbles and have taken to your bed in despair. It means that you're doing the smart thing in having a power nap.

Low mood – or is it depression?

If you feel exhausted on a regular basis, or feel suddenly incapable of doing your usual job, caring for your family or seeing your friends, things may be more serious. You may be suffering from a depressed mood, and if you can you should try to discuss this with a friend, counsellor or doctor. Weepiness is a common symptom of hormonal fluctuation at all stages in a woman's life: we all remember PMS outbursts, pregnancy mood swings, or baby-blues. But deep sadness associated with personal negativity, a feeling of failure, of intense dislike for oneself, may be difficult to manage. It's important to notice the difference between reacting to a sad situation and experiencing something deeper: weeping uncontrollably because you've locked yourself out of the house, for example, compared to weeping uncontrollably because you just can't face getting out of bed.

Many women are reluctant to discuss feelings of deep sadness, misery, loss of energy or a sense of worthlessness around the time of menopause, because they feel that either they will be fobbed off as hormonal, or offered hormone replacement without consideration of the real emotional situation; or they may assume that these intense feelings are just part of menopause and therefore have to be tolerated. They don't.

How do you know the difference between low mood and depression? Low mood is basically what doctors call the *feeling*, or the way you might present when you are suffering from depression. It is just what it sounds like: a mood that is low. But a mood can be temporary, or a reaction to a situation. In the worldwide recession of the current decade, many people have suffered from low mood, but this does not mean that they are ill, or not functioning normally. In the aftermath of a tragedy, or a loss, or during a time of personal suffering such as experiencing pain or relationship breakdown, it would be very reasonable to experience a low mood. And in these sorts of situations you might be very aware of your mood, but you will feel fairly comfortable discussing it with others, and you might also be aware that it will not last. You will feel better when you go on holidays, you will get over him, you can look forward to the weekend when the trials and tribulations of work are over for a while. Low mood can be persistent and difficult to shake, so that even if you want to cheer up you can get into a spiral of negative thinking, and this can easily be mistaken for major depression. However, doctors usually check for certain specific signs and symptoms that signify depression, as opposed to a temporary low mood.

If you are feeling depressed

If you consult with your doctor about your feelings of depression, she will probably ask you most, or at least some, of the following questions:

- Are you having trouble sleeping? Do you wake regularly during the night, or early in the morning, and are unable to get back to sleep?
- Have you lost your appetite, or are you eating more than you usually do without actually feeling hungry?
- Have you gained or lost significant weight?
- Have you lost interest in sex and relationships? Friendships? Family?
- Can you look forward to things – parties, weekends, holidays? Or are you finding it impossible to relate to loved ones and friends?
- Do you ever actually wish that you were dead, or think about ending your life?

If you were to answer 'yes' to the question on suicide, most doctors would try to find out if you have actually considered how you would plan to end your life. Do please talk to your doctor immediately if you ever feel like harming yourself, if you feel that others would be better off if you were dead, or if you wish that you could end it all. These are serious symptoms of depression and must be treated.

Treatments for depression

There is no stigma attached to asking your doctor for help in coping with depression. Your doctor will probably be grateful that you have mentioned it, and relieved that you are wise enough to seek medical help.

You may choose a drug-free treatment for depression, and most studies of antidepressants versus psychotherapy show that counselling and other therapies are just as effective in treating mild to moderate depression as are pharmaceuticals. Many GPs are now trained in cognitive behavioural therapy (CBT), psychotherapy, neuro-linguistic programming (NLP) or counselling, or can refer you to someone who can help you to cope with the changing patterns of persistently negative feelings and thoughts.

Antidepressant drugs work by altering the hormonal balance in your brain. Serotonin is the brain's chemical messenger that allows emotional activity to be normal, appropriate and responsive. Serotonin is secreted and received by cells during everyday emotional activity such as stress or worry, sadness, or other complex mental activities that require a lot of thought and cerebral attention. The more stress you are exposed to, mentally, the more serotonin your brain needs to secrete in order to allow neurones in the brain to respond to this stress: in other words, serotonin is a signal to the brain to 'up its game'. Serotonin is destroyed once it has been secreted by the cells, and therefore levels of serotonin can become rapidly depleted during periods of high stress.

Low levels of serotonin disturb sleep, mood and emotional responsiveness. Most modern antidepressant drugs work by eliminating the brain's natural ability to break down these hormonal chemical messengers, and this allows your brain cells to bathe in serotonin for longer, so that they can receive positive messages and do their work.

Some herbal remedies, such as St John's wort, have the same effect on serotonin. Cod liver and fish oil are thought to have a positive effect on serotonin levels in the brain, as is sunlight and vitamin D production. Exercise increases serotonin levels naturally, as does sleep, rest and laughter.

The best method of keeping up your natural serotonin levels is to make sure you get enough sleep, get out in the sunshine, seek out things that make you laugh, and avoid stressful situations, negative people and causes of anxiety.

Investing in counselling or therapy can be a wise and healthy way to spend your time and money. Whereas antidepressant drugs alter your mood and improve your energy while you are on them, therapy can help change your beliefs, values and attitudes to things in the longer term, so that you can prevent further episodes of depression or low mood.

Nobody's depression is without cause, and so if you can learn to cause yourself contentment and learn how to generate happiness, rather than allow depression to take over your mind, you can protect your mind and your body for the future.

Why does menopause affect the mood?

It may well be that the reduction of oestrogen affects the mood, or that it has a relationship with serotonin in the brain; the truth is, nobody really knows how. Hormones certainly do have a dramatic effect on mood, as you will remember from your pre-menstrual tension, when you felt weepy and forgetful in the couple of days before your period, when your levels of progesterone were high. Progesterone is often given as an artificial hormone in contraceptives like Mirena, or Implanon, and this has been associated with low mood. After menopause, when oestrogen levels are lower in the body, these hormonal changes may well be a cause for low mood. Among women who took hormonal replacement therapy during trials and in treatment, many reported dramatic improvements in their mood. But, equally, other women who also took HRT reported side-effects of weepiness, bloating and weight gain. Overall, studies have found that HRT had no particular effect on mood or depression in general, despite millions of women being prescribed it in the hope that they might find happiness.

The benefits of exercise on mood

One study has suggested that a tendency to develop psychological symptoms during menopause may be linked to factors such as level of education, high BMI and low physical activity. This is good news. If you are vulnerable to any of these risk factors, they are well within your control. Becoming a healthy weight is an available, instant mood lifter for pretty much any woman. Entering a learning environment or engaging in a course of study or extra-mural education in a subject that really interests you is a valuable, lifelong method of finding happiness. Exercise such as dance, yoga, Pilates, t'ai chi, boxing, running, swimming, cycling, has been shown to improve mood, not just during the period of exercise, but in general.

A large study in California looked at members of the population of Alameda County. The study examined three groups of people, who engaged in low, medium and high activity respectively, from the years 1965 to 1974, and found that the chances over 20 years of developing depression were highest in the low-activity group (1.75 times higher than in the high-activity group). A study in 2010, of 40,000 Norwegians, published in the *British Journal of Psychiatry*, found that being inactive outside the workplace doubled your risk of developing depression. Activity at work (such as lifting or cleaning) had no protective effect on depression.

Another study, which examined depressed people in 1999, divided 156 people with depression into three groups. One group did aerobic exercise, another took an antidepressant medicine, and a third took the antidepressants and took exercise. After 16 weeks, all had improved, but those who did aerobic exercise improved as much as those who had taken the antidepressant medicine. Furthermore, a follow-up study found that the positive results of exercise lasted longer.

Summoning up the energy to exercise when you are depressed can be a struggle, so start small and frequent. A quick walk around the block every night is a great start, if you've been very lethargic. Then start to timetable in a regular daily 30 minutes (minimum) of exercise that is aerobic: walking, cycling, running, swimming, dancing, boxing, or any contact sport.

Is work making you unhappy?

Menopause may well be a time to rethink your work situation and consider a change of pace. The early signs of ageing that you are noticing in your body are a prompt to you to take stock. Think about starting to put your self – your physical health, your mental health and your feelings and emotions – first, before your work, career and finances. It's a cliché to say that being healthy is much more important than being well-off, but it's quite true, and no career is worth making yourself ill or stressed for.

For older women success at work may bring related problems, such as struggling to keep up with younger colleagues, disguising signs of ageing, and trying to beat the looming spare tyre by desperate dieting with its endless cycle of hunger and guilt. Exhaustion and burn-out can result. The pull of the family on your working life is much stronger for women than for men. When offered big career opportunities or challenges in their mid-life, men are rarely plunged into despair at the thought of it!

Menopause, as I've stressed so far, is a time for change and you may need to examine how hard you are working and whether or not this is suiting your body at this time.

- Are you enjoying your job? Are you really feeling fulfilled and having fun? Or do you dread Mondays, struggle to keep up, have rows with colleagues, feel insecure, with too much pressure and responsibility?
- Are you using the time that you have, now that your children are more independent, to do things for yourself and at your own pace, rather than run around after their schedule all day long?
- Are you organizing your working day well, so that it's productive, by factoring in periods of rest, making time for proper meals, or streamlining your job description to ensure that it suits your changing life? Or are you slumping in the afternoons, struggling to get finished by 5 o'clock, and always missing deadlines?
- Are you making time to exercise? Or are you gradually gaining weight, feeling tired and becoming stiffer in the joints? Are you making time to enjoy your friends, lovers, hobbies, family?

- Are you enlisting help when you need it or are you still doing everything at home? Sometimes it's a good investment to pay someone to do a job you find difficult to fit in – ironing, cleaning, shopping, even domestic paperwork – so as to free up time and energy for yourself, which you can spend studying, playing, concentrating on your job, spending time with a loved one, or exercising more.
- Most of all, are you pencilling in your 'me-time' every day? 'Me-time' rarely just falls into your lap. You may have to schedule it. Is there space in your diary every day for time that is just yours?

According to Princeton University, a big trigger for unhappiness is commuting, especially if it takes more than an hour to get to work. America's 'happiest town' is San Luis Obispo in Northern California. In 1970 the town made a decision to change the environment so as to boost the happiness of its citizens. They simply made the sidewalks wider, which enabled the setting up of an infrastructure to make it easier to meet neighbours, sit in outdoor cafes, and walk or cycle rather than drive. Riding your bike instead of driving your car boosts your happiness by 50 per cent. And working for yourself instead of being an employee, even if this reduces your income by 50 per cent, increases your happiness by more than 50 per cent.

Studies of one million workers in the USA found that those in jobs where you have social interaction every day were the happiest. Fire-fighters, clergy, special education teachers and travel agents were occupations with the highest rate of happiness in America.

Princeton University also studied the relationship between happiness and money. It was found that happiness is connected with money up to a certain amount (at the time of the study, 2010, this was an income of around 75,000 dollars per year, per family – about £46,000). After this, working harder for extra income isn't worth it, as your unhappiness will increase. This is well worth knowing if you are planning a promotion, a career move, or a retirement! Making happiness your ultimate goal is likely to influence your decision-making, particularly when you are faced with big career opportunities or challenges.

Caring for others and bereavement

Mid-life is quite often a time when our parents may become ill or die. If you are in a situation of caring for them, you may feel that naturally you love your parents and are happy to do this for them, but you have been given a life-sentence of servitude to the elderly, sick and dying, only to be released from it all by another sentence of bereavement and sorrow in your own older age.

Losing your parents can come as a terrible shock, at any age, bringing with it very deep sorrow. It is important to try not to become overwhelmed by the death, or sickness, of a parent. If you are suffering a bereavement, or are coping with elderly or sick family, it is essential that you do not try to cope alone. Seek help and counselling during this difficult time. Hospices and hospitals often have experienced social workers, pastors and specialist nurses who can provide practical advice. Find a friend who knows what you're going through or who has had a similar experience to share the pain with. Bereavement counsellors are professionally trained to guide you through loss. Invest in this counselling as it will stand you in good stead in the future; it should help you to work through other griefs you may experience and with less of an impact on your own health and well-being.

Women in the menopause may have small children or grandchildren to care for, or teenage or adult children who bring their own sets of problems into our lives. With all the struggles in others' lives, it can be easy to forget to look after ourselves, and this can contribute to a low mood. Learning to be assertive is a good skill for any time, but particularly now, even if it takes a bit of practice. Take a few minutes to think about how to say things like: 'Well, I'd love to be able to help you with that, but I'm actually very busy at the moment/doing something else/very tired. Is there something else I could do for you instead, another time?' Building up confidence to say 'no' may save you hours, weeks, even years of anxiety and stress.

Women are much more likely than men to become carers of others. We tend not to put ourselves first for fear of being selfish. This means that we often leave care of ourselves and our own emotions and well-being until we are already exhausted or ill – by which time we are really suffering. Try to step off the treadmill before it's too late and you cause yourself long-term harm.

Depressive illness can be caused by doing too much, by becoming over-exhausted. Burn-out and tension, stress and worry, negativity and frustration all contribute. Untreated, depressive illness harms your physical health as well as your mental and spiritual health, limits your ability to enjoy life, and ultimately reduces your life expectancy. Do talk to your doctor if you are feeling genuinely depressed. Seek counselling and therapy in order to nip depression in the bud before it takes valuable years away from you.

Worry and stress

Worrying is a huge problem for women and is very strongly linked to low mood and depressive illness. Many women are chronic worriers. If you're worried about how much you worry, you're definitely not alone! So here is a strategy that will definitely help.

Allow yourself a certain amount of time – up to an hour – of solid worrying every day, at a pre-decided time. For example, if you find that you normally lie awake at night worrying, decide that instead you are going to worry for exactly one hour tomorrow at three o'clock in the afternoon. So, at three o'clock tomorrow afternoon you are going to clear your desk, get your worry beads out and do your worrying properly. Promise yourself that you will worry, really worry, for a whole hour, at three o'clock tomorrow afternoon.

Stress can affect you emotionally and physically. If you are experiencing acute stress, try this strategy. Step away from the environment in which you feel the stress and find a place to be alone and quiet. If you're driving, stop the car and pull over. If you're at work, take a break and leave the office if you can. If you're at home, go into another room or outdoors. Wherever you are, stop what you are doing completely, and take a long, deep breath and breathe out very, very slowly. Repeat this breathing several times, until you feel calm.

Think back to a time when you were very, very powerful. A time when you felt you could do anything. When you felt like a complete success. Visualize this time. Now close your eyes and put yourself right back into the experience. Where were you? Who was there with you? Listen to the voices, notice the background noises, remember what you were wearing, your perfume, what people said to you, and what you looked like. How pretty you looked. How smiley you felt. How amazing you were. Get yourself right back into this very state. Then, anchor this state by squeezing a knuckle or a fingertip – something that nobody will notice if you do it again. Now, when you have to go back into that stressful situation, fire your anchor to feel powerful again.

Ideas to increase happiness

Get to know your neighbourhood

Research at Harvard University and the University of California, San Diego found that having a friendly neighbour increases your happiness by 34 per cent. Getting to know your neighbours, 'living' in your neighbourhood, is good for you. Taking part in community activities, going to the local library rather than buying online books, patronizing local businesses, sending your kids to local schools, seeking out after-hours activities (classes, hobby groups, exercise groups) in your neighbourhood, all are likely to increase your personal happiness.

Double your money or double your fun

Studies of happiness at Harvard also found that becoming a member of a club where you have to show up at least once a month can have the same effect on your happiness as doubling your income. Most women have spent their whole adult lives building a career and caring for a family and have never found the time to join a club or develop a hobby. Making time for fun is something that many women find difficult to contemplate, but it is more important than any other intervention you could choose at this time in life.

Shopping for clothes or decorating your house can be a great source of fun. But research from the University of Colorado and Cornell University shows that buying new things or changing your surroundings will make you happier only temporarily – for up to about nine months – thereafter, the impact reduces. The effects of spending your money on having an experience – learning a new skill, joining a club, having a holiday, learning an instrument – last much longer.

Mindfulness

You can protect yourself against depression by becoming mindful. Mindfulness is a theory of self-care of the mind, derived from the traditions of meditation, retreating from the environment into yourself, to the here and now.

Negative states are associated with the past or the future. You may feel sad or humiliated, grief-ridden or rejected, guilty or hurt; these feelings are always connected with something that has happened in the past. Equally, you may feel anxious, fretful or worried, nervous, dreadful or afraid; these are all states associated with thoughts about the future.

Being mindful means that you are present in the moment. You are not leaving your mind in the past, or projecting into the future. You are simply here, in the moment. Learning to become mindful means adopting a habit of associating yourself with your present. Ask yourself the following.

- Where are you now? At this present moment? Are you sitting down? Where are you sitting?
- What does it feel like – the physical presence of your sitting, in this room, reading this book? Are you aware of your body, touching the pages of the book, listening to the slight rustling of the paper? Can you hear sounds – wind blowing, music in the background, traffic noise, city life, country birdsong?
- Is there a soft seat underneath you? Where are your feet? Your hands? Your neck? Take a moment to become aware of your body, and all its small movements.
- What is your breath doing? Spend a moment simply observing your breath entering and leaving your body, your chest rising and falling, your tummy rising and relaxing, your shoulders releasing as each breath enters your chest.
- Acknowledge this present moment, and the sensations you have in your body and in your mind, and be grateful for it. If there is worry there, acknowledge it. Say hello to it. Then let it go. You can return to it later. If there is fear or anxiety somewhere in your body, acknowledge that and let it go too. For the moment, you are only going to notice what is present in your body, and in your awareness of the here and now.

Zoning out like this into a meditative state allows you to become present to yourself, simply acknowledging the universe in which you exist at this moment.

Every day, ask yourself, 'How am I?' Just notice 'how' you are. 'I am stressed.' 'I am lonely.' 'I am worried.' 'I am happy.' 'I am optimistic.' 'I am tired.' 'I am interested.' 'I am alert.' Just notice your state, and acknowledge it without judging it. This is a very powerful habit to get into and has been shown in research to be strongly protective of your mood and resourcefulness.

We can't control time, and we can't control past or future events; we can only be mindful of the present. Mindfulness takes practice, preferably every day. Pencil in five minutes each day to start with; eventually you could work this up to half an hour, which will keep you healthier and happier for life.

The benefits of silence

Do you make time for silence? Harvard University found that just ten minutes of silence each day increases your happiness. Ten minutes isn't a huge amount of time! But it adds up, and provides you with value over your lifetime. Start with one minute, and build up towards ten; you could increase it to 20 or even 30 minutes as you get used to the positive effects.

Mindfulness (see above) is proven to help in personal development, in workplace relationships, in family relationships and in management of stress and depression. You can do a formal psychotherapeutic course in mindfulness practice or meditation, or, having become aware of the idea and theory of it, begin yourself to incorporate its principles into your daily life. So much of what we are encouraged to worry about are matters of the future and the past – just switching on the news reminds you of this, as the newsreader trawls through a list of woes of the world. Mindfulness is a habit that is the complete opposite of stress, and therefore it is a valuable resource that you can build into your life; it will strengthen your life and your emotional well-being into the future.

Find time to be alone and spend it wisely

Finding time to be alone can be very difficult. But it's not impossible – could you fit an hour for yourself every so often into your schedule? If you are running busy domestic days with play dates and after-school activities, or a busy office like clockwork, you may have to work at fitting in your 'me-time'. You may find this hour more easily if you timetable it; an hour spent as you would like, ideally each day but at the very least once a week, will be beneficial for your emotional well-being. Many women use the beauty salon or the bath-tub for this 'me-time'. Hygiene is important for your self-esteem. What about the internet café, the library, the cinema, university, night-school, or other public institution? Being alone can mean time to treat your body, but don't forget to nourish your mind.

Time spent alone can easily slip into a time of worry, fretting and planning furiously for the days and weeks ahead. This is where it is so important to be mindful. Going to a yoga class can help with mindfulness and meditation. Each yoga session ends with a meditation that you can repeat yourself at home. Yoga is proven in studies to treat depression effectively.

Or you could listen to a piece of music that's new to you. Just listen, really listen. Music is proven in studies to heal the troubled mind. Dancing to music is even better.

Learn to practise body-scanning. Either lie down or sit in a chair, quite still, with your eyes closed, then start to scan your body from the toes up, through every muscle and joint in the body. Notice where there is tension or tightness, and let it go, loosening and opening up so that you feel every bit of tension leave the body and allow yourself to relax completely, just observing your breathing.

A change for the best?

You may think of your menopause as a perfect storm of intense bodily and spiritual change. What happens as a result of the way you behave during this storm may affect your happiness for the rest of your life. You may throw all caution to the wind, and enter this storm clinging to your old, youthful habits, running out into the fray in a thin cotton frock and a pair of sandals, and spend the next ten years regretting your ill-thought-out venture, or you could take up the gauntlet and ride the storm magnificently in the most elegant rain-gear, emerging from the great adventure invigorated, inspired and made strong.

Consider asking yourself whether there are changes you could make to your life that would have a long-term effect on your happiness and emotional well-being. Look at the following list for ideas.

How are you living your life right now?

- Are you doing a job that you love, feel inspired by, and which satisfies your intellectual as well as financial needs?
- Do you give yourself enough time? Do you get ready in a calm way in the morning, with time to choose your clothes and jewellery, make a packed lunch or have a nutritious breakfast, or perhaps enjoy a quiet coffee in the garden before going to work – or are you frantically racing out of the door, buying a pastry to eat on the tube, racked with guilt?
- Could you have a bath in the mornings instead of a shower, giving yourself a little luxury time, ten minutes of calm and me-time, before work?
- Could you walk to the office, instead of using transport, so as to have an hour to think in the fresh air before the day begins?
- Are you filling your days with activities that excite you, that make you feel important and loved, or are you trapped in a domestic situation that's boring or lonely?
- Could you change some of this so that you have something good to look forward to each day?
- If you work from home, are you organizing your day so that household tasks don't just run into one another – are you finding time to exercise, to be in your garden or the local park? Are you eating proper meals and having regular work breaks?
- Are you finding time for a hobby?
- What is your passion? Are you finding time to be creative? Do you play an instrument/paint/write/garden, or make home crafts or DIY?

- Are you able at the end of each day to be alone for a while, either in the house in a quiet room or outdoors walking, gardening, playing a game – time during which you can completely switch off your mind from work and responsibilities?
- Are you making time to play? Play is thought of as being the most important way in which we exercise our minds, and an important route to relaxation, cognitive ability and relief from stress. Children are never stressed – and they play all day. Adults, especially women, are generally stressed and they rarely play! Puzzles, musical instruments, sports, video games – if you have grandchildren, or even teenagers, opportunities for these should come easily. (There is more about this in Chapter 8.) Joining others at play builds relationships. Playing with your partner is a huge relationship healer – chess, tennis, ping-pong, snooker, video games, basketball. Or sing together or play/learn a musical instrument.
- Who are you? Doctor, lawyer, retail worker, waiter, train driver, administrator, teacher, nurse? Mother, sister, lover, wife, grandmother, painter, tennis player, fisherwoman, friend? Thinking about your identity, about your purpose in the world, and which of your many roles is most important to you, helps you to focus your direction as you manoeuvre through the storm.
- What are you looking forward to tomorrow?

Two important things to remember, every day

- Other people's heads are far too wretched a place in which to leave one's sense of happiness (Schopenhauer).
- Think of something you were really stressed about ten years ago. It will make you smile. Remember that in ten years' time, you'll definitely be laughing about this too.

Symptoms of ageing were what I felt, really. Some loss of self-confidence, and the future seemed a bit bleak – I felt 'less empowered' at work, and that I was visibly ageing, and a bit sad that our children were growing away from us. But this was just because they were becoming independent, and I felt less needed. I didn't really understand their needs.

The lack of periods is the only good thing really – however, I do realize that self-obsession was counterproductive, so I hopefully will able to bounce back.

My biggest problem is feeling 'past it' (physically ageing, unglamorous) – how pathetic! As I grow older, I realize that I also feel a bit wiser, though.

There's no solution yet found to ageing, but I did more exercise, started having regular hair-styling, facials, also changed my job (not really for the better) but I suppose I had to expand my knowledge base and did new courses, sat exams (very difficult! – but so, so worth it).

My advice to other women is to address your physical and mental health and well-being, expand your interests, and don't whinge (especially to your family). It's very important to be smiley and interested in your friends, family, new acquaintances, and you reap the benefits of their interest and helpfulness. There's nothing so rewarding as feeling of value to others.

5

Preventing osteoporosis

Bones and bone turn-over

Throughout life, the substance of our bones is constantly being removed and replaced. Millions of tiny bone remodelling units are found on the surfaces of all our bones. Normal, healthy bone tissue is a hard structure; the cells contain calcium, the mineral that makes the cells tough. The amount of calcium found in a bone cell is what determines the density of the bone, and how strong it is, and it is what shows up on an X-ray of the skeleton. Bone mineral density declines as we grow older; low bone mineral density – osteopenia – can occur before the menopause, and other diseases and states of ill-health can cause low bone density. Osteopenia and osteoporosis (where the bone is so low in density that it has become porous and completely demineralized) are not confined to women.

Bone cells have what is thought of as a kind of turn-over of calcium during life. Calcium is absorbed from the diet and taken up into bone cells, enmeshed throughout the bony tissue; these cells mature and are gradually removed from the bone to make room for new bone cells growing up from the inside. The calcium is recycled back into the bloodstream, or resorbed, released by the outer cells of the bone tissue. There are three kinds of bone cell: osteoblasts, osteocytes and osteoclasts.

- Osteoblasts are the stem cells for the bone. They are responsible for taking up calcium from the blood and mineralizing the bone tissue with it. They are young cells, which mature and then turn into osteocytes.
- Osteocytes are the substance of the bone, and are cells matured from osteoblasts. They contain calcium and form the structure of the bone.

- Osteoclasts are the most mature of the cells, and are responsible for turning the calcium back out into the bloodstream again.

So a bone is a living tissue, in which the cells are constantly taking in calcium, turning it into structure for hard bone, and then dumping it back out into the bloodstream, pretty much the way the skin turns over nutrients from the bloodstream internally, works outwards, and eventually sheds.

This turn-over of bone is essential for strong, fracture-resistant bones; the cells are continually replaced in order to keep the bone supple and strong. This constant resorbtion or turn-over of calcium and bone cells is what rapidly diminishes after menopause.

But bone growth starts to settle down in our early twenties, of course. We don't grow in height after the age of 18–21. So although bone is constantly resorbed and rebuilt during life and the turn-over continues, the rate at which bone turns over diminishes from our twenties on. A bone that is broken or fractured will heal at any age in life; bone knits together again after a fracture, as the cells reach out to each other and reunite in order to form a new bony matrix, no matter what. But, this matrix requires a healthy amount of calcium, and a rapid rate of growth of bone cells from osteoblasts into osteocytes and then osteoclasts. This rate of turn-over is about six weeks in young adults, and about three weeks in children. But in older adults it can be 12 weeks or longer. The cells just don't turn over as quickly.

Factors affecting bone turn-over

Bone mineral loss can occur in women before the menopause, and in men; it can be affected by nutrition, illness, immobility, vitamin D deficiency, steroids, or disease of the parathyroid glands, which stimulate the bone to absorb calcium from the blood.

Some women have very little bone mineral loss after menopause. However, on average, in the years just after menopause, bone mineral loss is about 2 per cent per year and thereafter there is generally a steady slow bone loss of about 0.5 per cent per year. The age at which a woman actually develops osteoporosis or has bones that have lost calcium to the extent that they are now a fracture risk depends on what her bones were like before this loss began.

There is a time in our early twenties when we are at our 'peak bone mass'. Factors affecting bone mass in the twenties include the following.

- Calcium in the diet is essential in childhood and throughout life to stock up healthy bone. Diets low in calcium (lacking in dairy products) are associated with bone mineral loss.
- Vitamin D is needed to absorb calcium into bone. Vitamin D is only available from exposure to sunshine, although some dietary intake helps. Insufficient sunshine in childhood causes vitamin D deficiency or rickets (weak bones).
- Exercise stimulates blood supply and turn-over of bone. If bones are 'rested' too much, they are not stimulated to grow new cells and replace old, damaged ones. The rate of calcium resorbtion becomes slow, and not enough calcium is laid down into the matrix of the bone.
- A history of smoking is associated with future osteoporosis, leading to the theory that cigarette smoke affects calcium resorbtion and bone.
- Contraceptives based on progesterone, such as depot progesterone injections, are associated with loss of bone, because these are steroids that affect the resorbtion of calcium in bone.
- Steroids taken for asthma or other diseases cause demineralization of bone.

It has been found that African women tend to have higher bone mass and fewer fractures than Caucasian women, whereas Asian women tend to have lower bone mass, but also fewer fractures. This may reflect lifestyles and habits, such as exercise, smoking and drinking, of different groups of women, as well as their differing diets.

Women who had a poor diet in childhood, and sedentary habits in their twenties, who also smoke, never achieve peak bone mass. If you think you fit into this bracket, you should consider having a DEXA scan (see below), preferably in your forties, to check the mineralization levels of your bones.

Fractures – what's the risk?

Risk of fracture as a result of bone mineral loss increases with age. A white woman over the age of 50 has a 15 per cent risk of a hip fracture during her lifetime, which usually occurs before the age of 70. But she has a 40 per cent risk of at least one spinal fracture in her lifetime, and a 15 per cent risk of a wrist fracture; and many of these fractures occur in women before the age of 60. After a hip fracture, about two-thirds of women never regain their pre-fracture levels of function and independence. One in five women with a hip fracture die within a year of that fracture.

> I tripped and fell at the age of 46 and broke my wrist. It was an awful shock. It never occurred to me that I could have osteoporosis. I thought that only happened to old ladies! But because of the fracture my doctor suggested a bone scan and they found that my bones were so thin I was like a 90-year-old! I'd smoked all my adult life, though, lived on black coffees and never exercised. It was a real wake-up call. I force myself to the gym now but it's very difficult after a lifetime of bad habits. I did quit smoking and I take calcium, but I just wish I'd known about all the risks earlier.

What can I do to lower my risk?

These figures are pretty terrifying! Start, preferably in your forties, by discussing with your doctor your bone health, and examining your risk factors. A thorough assessment of whether or not you are at risk of osteoporosis or osteopenia should include the following.

- *Your weight.* High BMI and low BMI are both associated with osteoporosis. Rapid weight loss is particularly a risk.
- *Height measurement as a baseline.* Future height loss of over 3 cm suggests spinal or vertebral fractures.
- *Bone marker blood and urine tests.* These are not diagnostic tests but can be useful as a baseline for evaluating future treatments and interventions.
- *Bone scans.* The gold standard for the diagnosis of osteoporosis is a bone density test of the hip or spine called a DEXA scan (dual energy X-ray absorbiometry). Ideally both hip and spine

should be evaluated, because women with osteoporosis of the hip may not show osteoporosis of the spine, and vice versa. If only one site is scanned, in older women the hip is preferable; for younger women it is the lumbar spine area, because bone loss is visible earlier in the spine than in the hip. In the USA, bone densitometry is recommended for all women aged over 65; other countries don't measure this routinely unless there are additional risk factors.

Talk to your doctor about your risk factors. These include progesterone injectable contraception, a history of smoking, family history of fracture or osteoporosis, in your mother, aunts or sisters, lack of exercise especially in your twenties, a history of steroid medications during your teens or twenties, such as for asthma, a low calcium diet, any disease you have had that may have affected your ability to absorb calcium or vitamin D from the diet (bowel disease, coeliac disease, food intolerances, gall bladder disease and stones, anaemia).

Other diseases associated with osteoporosis in adults are Addison's disease, amyloidosis, anorexia, ankylosing spondylitis, chronic bronchitis, Cushing's syndrome, diabetes, endometriosis, gastric ulcer and operations, paralysis or immobility, multiple sclerosis, cancer, leukaemia, rheumatoid arthritis, and liver disease. Drugs and habits associated with osteoporosis include epilepsy treatments, cigarettes, alcohol, lithium, heparin, methotrexate, major sedatives, tamoxifen, steroids and retinol.

DEXA scans

The result from a DEXA bone scan compares your bone density to that of the average bone mineral density for healthy, young white women. The World Health Organization's definition of osteoporosis being present is a bone mass score that is at least two and a half times less than the standard deviation from the mean for a young adult reference sample. This means that they have examined the rate of spread of all the average bone density scores for a population of young healthy white adult women and found that within this range of scores, there's an average value and a measured, demonstrable *spread* or range of those normal values. They have calculated the rate of spread – in other words, the way in which normal bone mass differs from normal woman to normal woman. So if your bone mass is two and a half times less than would be expected in the average healthy white woman, then it is definitely low.

Osteopenia and osteoporosis – how exercise can help

Osteopenia means that your bone is demineralized, or low in calcium, which is reversible with treatment. Osteoporosis means that the skeleton is undergoing bony loss; although this is not reversible, you can make major changes to your lifestyle in order to protect your bones from further loss and fractures. Exercise is the key.

Although exercise in youth is most certainly proven to protect bones in the long term, exercise after mid-life and into later life has an essential effect of slowing bone loss. Clinical trials have shown that engaging in weight-bearing physical activity results in striking improvements in muscle strength and function and reduces risks of falls, injury and fracture by over 25 per cent even in the very elderly. Regardless of your affinity for exercise, if you do not regularly 'weight-train' your muscles, they deteriorate and weaken after middle age, very rapidly. Weak core muscles (the abdomen, internal pelvic and low back), quadriceps (thigh) and upper body, arm, shoulder and back muscles can cause big problems for middle-aged and older women, resulting in fatigue, loss of balance, trips and falls.

Most older women in western society do not have the upper body strength to lift their own body weight, or do a press-up. Test your upper body strength by seeing if you can lift yourself up from sitting in an armchair, using only your arms. If you cannot support your own body weight, you are at risk of not being able to get out of the bath one day! Start an upper-body strength programme now!

Weight-bearing exercises that are also aerobic include running, cycling, boxing, dancing, spinning, and heavy domestic housework. Swimming, Pilates, yoga and walking are not necessarily weight-bearing, and although these are fun activities and very beneficial they may not stress your muscles and bones enough to ensure the maximum stimulation to calcium resorbtion and strength of muscle to protect your bones.

Weight-bearing exercise for life

Resistance training using weight and gym machines has been shown in studies to promote bone health, increase muscle strength and improve bone density. You should always warm up first and alternate work between the arms and legs.

Begin with two leg exercises, followed by one upper-body exercise. Lift the weights slowly and take ten seconds in between each lift. Breathe in as you lift and breathe out as you lower the weight. To prevent injury, begin with weights that are 25 per cent of the maximum amount that you can lift. As you slowly progress, increase the weights to 85 per cent of your maximum. This should be done over three to four months.

Weight train every second day, taking a day's rest in between. Advice from a chartered physiotherapist with an interest in bone health may help you to keep motivated, prevent an injury and target your programme.

Personal training for bone health

Menopause is a time when you really need to take your exercise regime seriously. You may well have been an exerciser all your life, and any physical exercise is better than none. But tailoring your exercise regime to do the most for your bone health, your physical strength and fitness is a package that may need a professional guide. Many gyms provide a 'personal trainer' service and these trainers can be a resource in monitoring your fitness, weight and ability to use the equipment. A consultation with a physiotherapist is a useful start to a more therapeutic fitness and bone health programme, and if you are at risk of osteoporosis or have already been diagnosed with osteopenia, having a personal trainer who is a physiotherapist is a very useful investment now. Your physiotherapist can assess your risks, develop a weight and aerobic training programme that is tailored to your current needs and works with you over time, and is medically qualified to attend to any injuries you may develop.

Make your diet and lifestyle work for your bones

Enriching your diet in calcium makes a difference no matter what age you are, and if you have already been diagnosed with any arthritis, osteopenia or bone complaint you are advised to take a calcium supplement of 1,200 mg per day, as well as vitamin D. Adding calcium into your diet in the form of low-fat milk, yoghurt or cheese will cause no harm, and there are high levels of calcium in fish bones (as in sardines and anchovies), almonds and cruciferous vegetables (such as broccoli). Sunshine is essential for the body to make vitamin D, which is essential for the absorption of calcium into bone, so make sure to get out into daylight every day for an hour, even in winter.

6

Middle-age spread

Every woman gains weight after middle age because the metabolism slows down, and there is a tendency to eat more and exercise less. Many of us drive everywhere, and eat large meals because we have enough money to do so. We may be home-making or caring for others, which includes producing food pretty much every day. Being surrounded by food, spending hours in a kitchen, being the only one who does the weekly shop, all tend to increase the amount that we eat. The fact is that over 60 per cent of middle-aged women are now overweight in Britain and Ireland, as well as in the USA. This isn't just bad for our self-esteem or our vanity: it is bad for our health. Excess weight, as mentioned earlier, is known to be associated with breast cancer, and it is well known that it's also associated with heart disease, blood pressure, stroke and diabetes.

Attending to your weight at menopause could save your life.

Body mass index:
the medical standard of measurement

Body mass index (BMI) measures the relationship between your height and weight. So you can't run and you can't hide. Big-boned it ain't: BMI takes into account the exact size of your bones and calculates your ideal weight. The range is quite generous too, so if you are overweight on a BMI chart, don't avoid facing up to it. You are endangering your health and you should do something about it.

Recent studies of diabetics and those who are pre-diabetic, or overweight people who develop diabetes, have found that measuring the waist can accurately predict whether or not someone is at risk of developing diabetes. Women with a waist measurement of more than 32 inches, at any age, are assumed to be at risk. Do take this advice seriously, because even if you are able to tolerate the misery of the changing room or beachside when you are overweight, you will not enjoy losing a foot to diabetes. Measure your waist now. If it's over 32 inches, read on.

The body mass index (BMI) is a statistical measurement calculated from your weight and height. It's used to estimate a healthy body weight, based on how tall a person is. Body mass index is your weight (in kilograms) divided by your height (in metres) squared. There are many sites online that can calculate your BMI, or you can use a BMI chart (see Figure 1, opposite) or work it out for yourself.

$$BMI = \frac{mass\ (kg)}{height^2\ (m^2)}$$

It is estimated that 38 per cent of British and Irish women are overweight (have a BMI greater than 25), and 23 per cent are obese (BMI greater than 30). A BMI greater than 40 is called 'morbidly obese'. This means that your weight is a danger.

The relationship between death and body weight is a J-shaped curve, with a sharp increase in the risk of death, from all causes, when the BMI is over 30. However, the upswing of the curve starts at a BMI of 25. The risk of coronary artery disease increases three-fold in women with a BMI greater than 29, compared to those of a BMI of 21.

Big solutions to big problems

Drugs

If your BMI is greater than 30, see your doctor for advice. You need to be checked out for diabetes, blood pressure, and you may need blood tests, for instance for thyroid hormone level. Doctors are well trained in prescribing anti-obesity drugs, and if you are dangerously overweight this can sometimes be a good place to start, giving you the confidence to keep going. But these drugs mainly work by excreting extra fat from your bowel, so many women find these unacceptable, as the stools become fatty and foul-smelling.

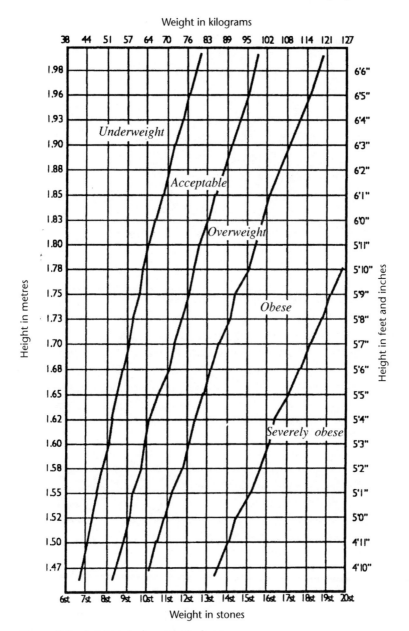

Figure 1 Body Mass Index (BMI) chart

Source Taken from Dr Robert Povey, Dr Claire Hallas and Dr Rachel Povey, *Living with a Heart Bypass*, London: Sheldon Press, 2006, p. 82.

Other anti-obesity drugs affect appetite. Because they all work via the central nervous system they have side-effects of nausea and drowsiness, and can affect your liver. Therefore anti-obesity drugs may be a good short-term measure, but ultimately you need a healthy eating plan for life.

Over-the-counter or on-prescription drugs can:

- increase fat loss (orlistat)
- decrease appetite (cannabinoids)
- increase fluid loss (diuretics)
- increase heart rate and metabolism (amphetamines, caffeine).

All drugs that have these effects will also have side-effects.

Surgery

Weight-loss surgery is sometimes recommended if you are morbidly overweight and incapable of making dietary and lifestyle changes. The results of this sort of surgery (stomach stapling, gastric banding, partial gastrectomy) are radical weight loss. But all these operations carry risks, from general anaesthetic, clots and infection, especially as surgery in obese people is so much more difficult for surgeons to perform. After surgery you will always have digestive deficiencies, and will have to take vitamin and mineral supplements for life.

Obesity surgery can cause weight loss by decreasing the size of your stomach so you feel full quicker, or by removing your ability to absorb the fat in your diet. The more sudden the weight loss, the more likely you are to have long-term side-effects from the surgery. For morbidly obese people, however, these operations can be life-saving.

Crash dieting

If you are very overweight, going on a reduced calorie diet can indeed seem like a crash for your body. Obese women may well be used to eating anywhere from 2,500 to over 4,000 calories per day, so reducing this to 1,500 or even 1,000 calories, which is what most diets recommend, can be sudden and difficult. However, if you are dangerously overweight, you need to rapidly lose weight too, and reducing calories is the most effective way to do this.

Do any celebrity diets work?

Studies have been done to see if any 'celebrity' diets work for long-term weight loss and diabetes control.

The Pritikin diet, a fat-free, whole-food diet that was very fashionable in the 1980s, loses weight quite rapidly but in the long term can be found unpalatable and difficult to maintain. The low GI (glycaemic index) diet is easy to follow long term but loses the least amount of weight; however, doctors do recommend it as safe, healthy, and suitable for women at risk of or who already have diabetes. The Hay diet, which involves food combining (in particular, not eating protein and carbohydrates at the same meal) is good for long-term weight loss but it's quite anti-social! Dieters are likely to lose weight, slowly, but then keep the weight off. You may find this a useful way of reducing calories without having to calculate or worry about them too much, and it's easy to organize what to eat.

Those following the Atkins diet (carbohydrate-free) have been shown to lose the most weight but they are also the most likely to 'relapse'. The theory of the diet is that the digestion of food itself causes the body to lose energy, which if not replaced in carbohydrates will automatically lead to the burning of fat. The problem is that eating a meal without carbohydrates can leave you feeling hungry as your body burns this fat! If you need to lose weight quickly, Atkins is easy to follow, and safe in diabetes as long as you don't eat too much fat, but it is not a balanced diet. It does not contain fruit, so you can become vitamin-depleted. A high protein diet can cause kidney problems and constipation, damaging your bowel, and people on such a diet may experience fatigue; the body can also become 'ketotic' or experience glucose starvation if starved of carbohydrates. If you are following this diet, try not to eat fatty meat and fried foods just because they are 'carb free': they are still bad for your heart! Instead, enjoy meals that are mostly based on vegetables, fish, eggs and chicken.

Healthy eating for life

The truth is that many dieters relapse and regain the weight they have lost, so we need an easy-to-maintain nutritional strategy for life. Middle age and menopause is the ideal time to take stock of your eating habits and see where you are making consistent mistakes. Consulting with a nutritionist will allow you to figure out what your ideal calorie intake should be, and to plan meals around that.

Balanced nutrition

A well-balanced diet means having meals in which 50 per cent of the calories are from carbohydrate-containing foods, less than 35 per cent from fats, and 12–15 per cent from protein. Contrast this with many 'meat and two veg' meals in which approximately 50 per cent of the plate is covered with protein, most of the other 50 per cent being carbohydrates smothered in fat.

The daily protein requirements of the average person are covered by about 1 gram per kilogram of body weight (higher for an athlete, perhaps 1.6 grams per kilo). This is equivalent, if you are 50–60 kilos in weight, of one meal a day with a piece of meat about the size of a deck of cards, and another with a slice of cheese or an egg. Dairy foods contain protein as well as calcium, but they are also mainly high in fat. If you are avoiding these in order to protect your weight, don't forget the risk of osteoporosis and osteopenia. If you are not eating calcium-containing dairy foods, take a supplement of 1,200 mg of calcium per day.

Carbs, sugar, and the glycaemic index

Not all carbohydrates are the same. There are simple, sugary carbohydrates found in sugar, potatoes, white rice and pasta, and these are rapidly converted to glucose in the small intestine, stimulating an insulin surge from your pancreas. These are what we call high GI foods: the glycaemic index is a measure that diabetologists have developed to describe the rate at which certain foods can be converted to glucose. Obviously, for diabetics, high GI foods are a no-no; as they are quickly converted to glucose, they cause a huge demand for insulin. High GI foods can be dangerous in the non-diabetic too. The sudden high in blood glucose, which occurs pretty much as soon as they are eaten, is soon followed, after the stimulation of the huge rush of insulin, by a rapid lowering of the blood glucose again. This process can cause 'dumping', the exhausted, low-energy feeling you get after a large, bread-filled lunch. And unless you are actively exercising as you eat this high GI food, the sudden rush of insulin forces the carbohydrate to be immediately converted into glycogen and stored as fat. Thus, not only is this huge energy meal no longer available to you to utilize, it is now sitting right on your hips.

Low GI foods, on the other hand, don't destabilize the blood sugar. They make the energy you have eaten in your food available to you by releasing small amounts of glucose into the bloodstream at a steady, low rate throughout the day, and allow you to feel satisfied and full and yet not exhausted after a meal. Doctors now recommend a low GI diet for all diabetics, and for non-diabetics who want to feel well and prevent weight gain.

Make the most of what you eat

Eating a balanced diet means that you should eat three meals a day, each of which contain less than 20 per cent protein, about 50 per cent carbohydrate, and the rest as vegetables, mainly low-calorie greens.

Of the 50 per cent carbohydrates, make the emphasis on low GI ones such as peas and beans, sweet potato or yams, brown rice or other whole grains, oatmeal, nuts and fruit, and avoid white rice, pasta, white bread or potato. If you are having potato, eat the skins as well, as this lowers the overall GI of the meal. If you are eating peeled potatoes, white rice or pasta, mixing this 50/50 with a green vegetable lowers overall GI.

Eating protein with carbohydrate for each meal (for example, whole-grain cereal with soya or cow's milk, or egg with wholemeal toast, cheese, tuna or chicken and salad sandwich on wholemeal bread with a piece of fruit, and lean fish with vegetables, brown rice and salad) means that you will feel satisfied afterwards. Always make sure to eat foods from both food groups with each meal, even at breakfast, or if it's just a sandwich.

Aim to eat as much raw food as possible: add things like salad, fruit, tomatoes, nuts, seeds, carrot, celery, radishes, avocado to every meal. Raw foods contain vitamins and antioxidants that fight cancer and cellular ageing, and help you prevent weight problems for life.

Try to eat different coloured fruits and vegetables; and mix white foods with green. So, if you are eating potatoes always have greens, such as salad, cabbage, broccoli, green peppers, as this will increase the nutritional value of the meal as well as lower the high GI effect of the potatoes. As for white rice or pasta, don't eat more than one handful in any one day, and always eat with green vegetables; this will also protect your liver.

Foods that have no nutritional value (and that people like to eat!):
- crisps
- pastry
- cake and biscuits
- sweets and chocolate
- fizzy drinks
- alcohol.

Comfort foods that are also nutritious treats:
None of these foods will cause you weight problems (provided you eat nuts in moderation) and they will satisfy a 'treat' need.
- bananas, mandarins, fresh pineapple, fresh strawberries, melon
- raw almonds, brazil nuts, hazelnuts
- smoked salmon
- hummus
- peanut butter
- avocado.

Tips:
- Fill your pantry with exotic fruits and nuts to snack on, or for an after-dinner sweet, to prevent sugar cravings.
- Munch raw carrot and celery with hummus as a snack instead of crisps.
- Drink a large glass of water before each meal, as this helps to prevent overeating.

Keep a food diary

Keeping a food diary for a couple of days can be a very revealing exercise – sometimes quite frightening! Having to record every morsel that you put into your mouth has a curiously steadying effect on what you eat. Most of all, you will quickly identify the problem foods that are causing you weight problems.

More than just eating habits

Research into obesity has revealed that no matter which way we spin it, most overweight people are fat because they eat too much. Too many calories, plain and simple. And, most people with a weight problem are in denial about what they eat. Having an honest conversation with yourself and your loved ones may help to identify what eating habits you could change. Start with your portion size: nobody needs seconds; and aim to eat only about two handfuls of food per meal, which is enough for an adult plateful.

Developing a regular exercise habit helps to increase your fitness and improve your metabolic rate, as fat is converted to muscle. Weight-bearing exercise is essential for women after menopause. But dancing, running, cycling, boxing, spinning, swimming lengths and fast walking are the best calorie burners. If you are out of the habit of exercise, start small and increase with small, daily goals. A ten-minute walk may seem a lot at first, but do ten minutes today, and tomorrow try 15. Increase when you feel ready, but most importantly, keep up a daily habit. This way you can build up to a regular 30-minute daily habit of vigorous calorie burning, rather than trying to do a full 30 minutes in one go from the very start.

Timetable this half-hour of exercise each day. It doesn't matter what you do, but make sure you have a time for it, and stick to it.

Plan your meals

Nourishing your body every day means that you need to take the time to plan your meals. A few simple rules make balanced meals easier.

- Something purple or red every day.
- Something green every day.

- Always mix white foods with green.
- Fish three times a week.
- A handful of seeds or raw nuts every day.
- Five portions of fruit and vegetables every day.
- Fresh water to drink before every meal.
- Foods from all three food groups at every meal.

What makes people fat? Studies of behaviour can tell us about the habits that make some people fat, and those that help to keep others slim.

Seven habits that fat people often have:

1 Driving a car.
2 Watching TV.
3 Eating late at night.
4 Having a main meal after 7 p.m.
5 Eating between meals.
6 Avoiding breakfast.
7 Socializing with alcohol.

If you regularly do any of these, you may have identified a fat habit that you can easily change.

Seven habits that slim people often have:

1 Goal-setting: knowing their weight, waist measurement, ideal weight.
2 Self-monitoring (keeping a food diary, calorie counting, using points system).
3 Eating correct portions, not having seconds (a portion of meat is 75–80 grams, a portion of cheese 25–30 grams; you don't need any more), and never eating more in one sitting than the amount of food that can be held in your two hands.
4 Eating a main meal in the middle of the day.
5 Always eating breakfast.
6 Cooking fresh, nutritious food, not relying on takeaways or ready meals.
7 Exercising every day for at least half an hour: walking, running, swimming, going to the gym, dancing, whatever gets the body moving.

7

What can I do to prevent cancer?

Cancer: be aware of the risks

With ageing, the increased risk of cancer is unfortunately inevitable. A third of all women develop cancer at some point in their lives, one in five develops breast cancer, and cancer is the cause of over a quarter of all women's deaths. Lung cancer is now the main cause of death from cancer in all women, although breast cancer is the most common woman's cancer. Lung cancer is, and has been since the 1950s, clearly associated with smoking, to such an extent that the government warns smokers on every pack of their likelihood to die. But we now know that women's therapeutic hormones, found in the pill and HRT, cause breast cancer. In fact, the incidence of breast cancer has risen dramatically over the last 30 years, coupled with the increase in uptake of contraceptive hormones and HRT. The regrettable fact is that the contraceptive pill and hormone replacement therapies are known, and have been since their original manufacture in the 1920s, to be associated with cancer, of the womb and the breast. But the vast majority of women who take these hormones, especially those of us who are or have been on the contraceptive pill, were never really made aware of the danger.

Doing research that proved these associations has not been easy. In fact, for doctors to try to expose the risks of the pill and HRT has been as controversial and irritating to the relevant industries as trying to expose the cancer risk of cigarettes was to Big Tobacco, back in the 1960s.

Sexual freedom is important, and for the majority of young women in need of birth control, advocating an end to the use of the oral contraceptive and a return to the risks of multiple, unwanted pregnancies would cause extreme hardship. But other lifestyle factors associated with freedom and independence for women appear to be associated with cancer too. The *British Journal of Cancer* published the finding that drinking more than one unit of alcohol per day increases your lifetime risk of developing breast cancer by almost 10 per cent. Yet no wine manufacturer is going to put a label on their best vintage, reminding women of their risk of breast cancer should they open up a bottle.

Warnings about women's risk of cancers seem to be restricted to daffodil brooch-selling, pink ribbons and beard-growing in November. If the manufacturers of these proven, carcinogenic toxins in our environment are not prepared to take responsibility for the cancer-producing effects of their drugs and lifestyle products, then all we can do for now is arm ourselves with the best possible knowledge and advice for a strategy for cancer prevention throughout our lives.

In general, women have always been much more likely than men to be aware of the relationship between lifestyle choices, the environment and health, and consequently be keen to make wise health choices. For example, although our consumption of fruits and vegetables has risen sharply since the 1980s, it did not rise significantly in men until the 'five a day' campaign, bearing out the theory that men respond better to simple, numeric messages about health, whereas women are more likely to research ideas about health gain. But the drive to give positive health messages for women has not been applied with the same levels of seriousness. Women's health messages aren't necessarily effective either, when framed in a childish way. Encouraging breast self-examination, for example, has not been shown in studies to have had any effect on breast cancer detection.

Women can no longer be fobbed off with simple, childish messages when it comes to wanting information about how to prevent cancer. We need better, more scientific, more meaningful information, so as to make well-informed, valuable decisions about the way to live our lives.

Genetic mutations and family history play an important part in women's cancer, and therefore women who have a close relative with breast cancer are now invited to be screened for cancer-risk mutation genes. However, the vast majority of breast and ovary cancers are not genetically linked. Only about 10 per cent of women's cancers are found to have a causative gene that can be identified. It is easy to feel as though one is bound to become a victim to cancer, and to live in terror of this pandemic disease that creeps up on women by stealth, and from which we seem to have no protection. Thankfully, some research is being done into lifestyle and cancer, and the known risks that are associated with weight, fat consumption, alcohol and other environmental factors are well within our control.

Cancer screening

Most western countries now have a well-organized screening programme for breast and cervical cancers. Sadly, there is no screening programme yet for ovarian cancer, although women are now asked about family history and can be screened for the associated gene. Ovarian cancer is, therefore, thought to be more lethal than breast or uterine cancer as it can go undetected for many years, before a woman notices any change to her health.

Being aware of the risks of ovarian and breast cancer in your family is a good place to start. Become aware of lifestyle measures (discussed later in this chapter): diet, alcohol, exercise. Have a yearly check-up for your breasts, and attend for a mammogram when you are called. Have a yearly bi-manual pelvic examination to examine your womb and ovaries, and go for your smear whenever your doctor or screening programme advises. Find out if you have had the HPV virus, which is known to be the cause of cervical cancer: a simple blood test can do this.

Cervical cancer

Screening – the smear test

A cervical smear test is a screening test for a woman's tendency to develop cervical cancer. But a screening test is not a diagnostic test. So having a screening test for cancer will identify two groups of women: women who need further testing because they might have cancer or might have a risk factor for cancer, and women who seem to have no need for further testing at this point in time. A positive smear means that the doctor has identified some cells that are 'dyskaryotic', or look abnormal. They might become cancerous, in the future. You will need another test, such as a biopsy or a colposcopy (examination with a camera microscope). A normal smear, on the other hand, means that no abnormal cells were found.

Screening, therefore, is quite a cumbersome procedure, depending on what you are looking for. However, ever since organized cervical cancer screening was introduced, in Scandinavia in the 1960s, the benefits have been obvious. The mortality from cervical cancer was reduced by 76 per cent in Iceland, and the incidence by 75 per cent in Finland. Now, all women over the age of 25 in the UK are invited for screening by the NHS, and evidence demonstrates that there is a clear reduction in deaths from cervical cancer due to this screening programme.

But is screening for cervical cancer enough? We now know that cervical cancer is caused by the HPV wart virus, and so young women these days are being vaccinated. Most probably in the future the smear test will be replaced with a virology blood test, and the need to have smears every five years will be no more; women who have had HPV will be identified and they alone will be smeared. In the meantime, you can have the blood test quite easily; if you have had a history of vulval or vaginal warts you should let your doctor or smear-taker know, as she will need to take more frequent smears.

I have had a 'recall' on my smear test – does this mean I have cancer?

In about 10 per cent of smear tests, the cells can't be seen clearly enough, so if you are recalled this may be the simple reason. In about another 10 per cent there is an abnormality, so you should most certainly have your repeat test done.

Of the women who are recalled for another test, over half (58 per cent) will have to have another smear test because of positive results. Of this group who have persistently positive smear tests, between 2 and 22 per cent are found to have pre-cancerous changes in the cells. If you have had a recall request on your smear, then, there is a slim chance that it is abnormal, so do go. But, in the vast majority of cases, the recall test is fine.

Does the cervical smear test pick up all cancers?

Cervical smear testing can pick up about 80 per cent of all cervical cancers, so this means that it misses some too. Therefore, do look out for other symptoms throughout life, especially after menopause.

Signs to look out for in detecting and preventing cancer

Bleeding between your periods or after your periods have finished (post-menopausal bleeding) is always abnormal and must be investigated. It doesn't always mean that you have cancer, but it must be checked out. Please talk to your doctor if you have any bleeding you're not sure about, and particularly after the age of 50. Discharge, especially if it is pink, or brown – in other words, not exactly bleeding but bloody-looking – is also abnormal and should be investigated. It may be caused by polyps, infection, or other non-cancerous reasons.

Painful deep sexual intercourse, pelvic pain, constipation or a sudden change in bowel habit, should be immediately investigated.

Any cystitis, urinary tract infection or urinary symptoms need some sort of medical attention. Simple cystitis should not need antibiotics unless there is proven bacterial infection, and should respond to cranberry products. Urinary tract infection or cystitis that does not respond to cranberry juice needs to have a sample sent to the lab. A dip-stick is not enough to diagnose the cause of the infection. If your doctor is treating your urinary tract infection with antibiotics, make sure you request a laboratory diagnosis. Always empty your bladder before and immediately after intercourse.

Breast cancer

For many decades, the most that the medical profession could come up with to prevent this disease, which was rapidly increasing in incidence, was to tell women to be 'breast-aware'. Well, which woman is not, at almost every moment of her life, breast-aware? Is it actually possible to get through a single day without being aware of one's breasts, and those of other women around you? At this time, I am counting my close friends, family members and neighbours who have had, still have, or have died of breast cancer. I have run out of fingers. I could not, in fact, be more aware of breasts.

Ask your doctor to examine your breasts regularly, and always get your doctor to immediately check if you feel any lumps, or notice any discharge or nipple changes. If you feel that there is something unfamiliar or not right in your breast, make sure that all your concerns have been answered, and seek a second opinion or a biopsy and ultrasound if you have a lump of any sort. Although most lumps are not cancer, this is not satisfactory as an explanation for any woman who feels there is a lump there, so make sure that you are satisfied that you have been thoroughly investigated, no matter what.

Being 'breast-aware' is clearly not enough to prevent or manage this pandemic disease among modern women.

Screening after menopause: the mammogram

The value of mammography, as a screening test for women aged over 50, has been assessed. In pretty much all trials mammography reduces death rates from breast cancer in all populations. Mammography is expensive, requires a high level of expertise, and exposes women to a dose of radiation that could be of itself harmful, and therefore for many decades doctors had mixed feelings about the value of screening all women for breast cancer. However, results from the original Swedish trials in mammography were quite clear. The researchers found that they could reduce death rates by 25 per cent from breast cancers if they screened all women over 50. The NHS now recommends three-yearly mammography to women aged 50–70. The value of picking up breast cancers in women younger than this is thought not to outweigh the harm caused by exposing women to radiation and the anxiety of the test.

Internationally, however, standards for screening differ and women are offered different services at different ages, depending on where we live. In 2009 the United States Preventive Services Task Force made new recommendations that mammography screening for women who are not at increased risk of breast cancer should be started at 40 years of age. The age range at which the NHS offers free screening is due to increase by the end of 2012 to include all women from age 47 to 73. In Ireland, where routine free screening was very lately developed, women are screened only between 50 and 64.

Sadly Ireland's success in preventing deaths from breast cancer lags far behind the USA and the UK.

If you've ever had a mammogram, you'll know that it is an uncomfortable test, and time-consuming. You have to go to a special mammography unit and have an X-ray, exposing your breasts to radiation. Most women welcome the invitation to mammography, though, despite it being a rather unpleasant process. An X-ray is taken of the breast, side on, during which the breast is compressed quite strongly between two heavy X-ray plates. This is likely to be painful, and so your doctor and radiographer will warn you that it is not pleasant. But it is brief!

The X-ray is then read by two radiology experts in breast cancer, to reduce the risk of mistakes. Two 'views' are taken at each appointment, and you are sent a written result. Some women will be 'recalled', and asked to have a follow-up appointment. This may involve an ultrasound, a further clinical (manual) examination, or a fine-needle biopsy. If there is a definite lump, you will probably be asked to have a surgical biopsy of this, under anaesthetic.

Mammography, like any other screening test, has false negative results. And many cancers present with an actual lump, especially in younger women who have not been routinely called for a screening mammogram. So, as said above, we also need to be (and are!) breast-aware, although self-examination is not enough to detect or prevent cancer.

I have been told I need 'further investigations' from my mammogram. Does this mean they have found a lump?

About 5 per cent of women who have had a screening mammogram will be called for 'further investigations'. After these investigations, a woman may be either (a) diagnosed with cancer, (b) diagnosed with a pre-cancerous lesion (ductal cardinoma in situ, or DCIS), which requires removal, (c) placed on an 'early recall' list, or (d) given the all-clear. 'Early recall' means that a woman is not sent the results of her test but asked to come back for a further test (before the next regular three-year screen). This usually means another appointment in six or 12 months.

About six in every 1,000 women *screened* turn out to have cancer. About 11.6 per cent of all women who are sent for further investigations will turn out to have cancer. In other words, about 5 per cent of all screened women are recalled, and of those, about one in every ten actually have cancer. The other nine of the ten are given the all-clear.

The majority of cancers that are picked up through screening are non-invasive or micro-invasive cancers, or are very small in size. These cancers can mostly be taken out by just removing the lump, although this depends on the position of the cancer in the breast.

Not all cancers need to be treated with chemotherapy or hormone-blockers. And not all breasts need to be completely removed. Cancer treatment, genetics and surgery are improving rapidly. New treatments develop every year, with better side-effect profiles and long-term results. Oncology treatment is very specialized and well integrated with psychological, social and other well-being services.

The death rate from breast cancer is reduced by 26 per cent in women who have had screening.

Family cancers and genetic testing

Two genetic mutations, known as BRCA 1 and BRCA 2, are known to result in a lifetime risk of breast cancer of up to 80 per cent, and of ovarian cancer of up to 60 per cent. These genes are inherited in a dominant fashion, so if you have a sister, mother, aunt, or other close family relative with breast or ovarian cancer, try to find out if she has been tested for the gene. Then have the test yourself, and if you have daughters they can be tested too.

The results may be surprising. Although the gene is dominant, it has what is known as 'variable penetrance', which means that not all females with the family gene will inherit the cancer risk. Many women will find that although their mother has the gene, they themselves have not inherited it.

Of all cancers, about 5 per cent are caused by the high risk gene. However, if you have the gene your risk of developing cancer at a young age is so high that surgeons are now advocating preventive, prophylactic mastectomy and bilateral oophorectomy in women who test positive for this family cancer gene.

Lifestyle factors and the prevention of cancer

The World Cancer Research Fund (WCRF) confirmed in a report that there are some very important links between diet and lifestyle factors and cancer, including breast cancer. The report is a summary of findings from over 7,000 research studies from around the world. Since so many studies were closely reviewed, the findings are believable and hard to debate.

Keeping slim turned out to be one of the most important things a woman, or a man, can do to lower the risk of cancer. Because the hormones that can influence breast cells (oestrogens) and the development of breast cancer are made in fat tissue, excess body fat can increase a woman's chance of developing breast cancer after menopause.

Here are some of the report's most important recommendations:

- Maintain the body weight that's ideal for you. Weigh yourself, find your BMI and stick to a BMI that's under 25.
- Eat a diet low in fat and rich in fruits and vegetables. Coloured fruits and vegetables contain anti-cancer properties, known as antioxidants, which fight cancer-change in cells.
- Avoid red and processed meats, simple carbohydrates (sugar, sweets, white bread, cakes), and salt.
- If you have a baby, breastfeed for at least the first six months.
- Do not smoke.
- Avoid alcohol.
- Engage in regular exercise of moderate intensity.

Alcohol and cancer

The Million Women Study in the UK found that women who drank were more likely to develop several types of cancer, including breast, compared to women who didn't drink. The higher cancer risk was seen *even in women who regularly drank only small amounts of alcohol.* The researchers estimated that *the accumulated effect of each alcoholic drink per day increases breast cancer risk by about 12 per cent.* So, compared to a woman who doesn't drink, a woman who has one daily drink has about a 12 per cent risk of breast cancer; a woman who has two drinks a day has about a 24 per cent risk of breast cancer.

Researchers don't completely understand why drinking alcohol seems to increase breast cancer risk. Other studies have shown that hormone-receptor-positive breast cancer is the type most affected by alcohol. Oestrogen can cause hormone-receptor-positive breast cancer to develop, and alcohol can increase the amount of oestrogen in a woman's body. Therefore this increase in oestrogen may be part of the reason for the link between alcohol and breast cancer risk.

The Million Women Study also found direct links between taking artificial oestrogen pills and breast cancer. The oral contraceptive pill which contains oestrogen slightly increases the risk of breast cancer, while hormone replacement oestrogen (HRT) definitely increases the risk of breast cancer.

The advantages of soya products

Breast cancer surgeons nowadays feel that soya is more breast-friendly than dairy. Soya foods contain phyto-oestrogens, or plant-based oestrogens, which are thought to block the body's response to the cancer-causing natural oestrogens that every woman has. However, this cancer-preventing role of soya hasn't been replicated in studies, and is based on population studies in Asian women who have low rates of breast cancer compared to western women. Soya (tofu, miso, soy milk) can, however, help with symptoms of HRT for women who don't want to take oestrogen and therefore it could definitely be said to be more 'breast-friendly'. And soya in the diet reduces the risk of osteoporosis after middle age.

Aluminium in deodorant: is it a risk?

Although plenty has been written about the assumed link between the aluminium contained in some deodorants and breast cancer, when it comes to scientific proof the jury is still out. But many women feel happier using aluminium-free deodorant. Aluminium is excreted in breast milk, however, and therefore we do know that breast tissue has an affinity for this metal. Shaving the skin in the armpit increases the risk of absorbing antiperspirant products into the glands.

Seven hours a week of vigorous exercise

Much research has shown a link between regular, moderately intense or vigorous exercise and a lower risk of breast cancer. While less intense exercise can benefit general health, research suggests that lower intensity exercise doesn't really bring down your cancer risk. A study from the National Cancer Institute in the USA found that only vigorous exercise was linked to a lower risk of breast cancer in post-menopausal women, and only when that exercise was done from mid-life onwards. Post-menopausal women who had maintained more than seven hours a week of higher intensity activity over the ten-year period prior to entry into the study were 16 per cent less likely to develop breast cancer. But reductions in risk were not achieved with light activity, or with more intense exercise earlier in life. Therefore, it's important to exercise vigorously during and after middle age.

Sarah's story

Sarah had a dynamic career as a musician and was very slim and fit. After she married, however, she gained a lot of weight and by her forties was quite obese. Having had two children, she felt sure that middle-age spread was just a fact of life. She also enjoyed plenty of wine, and had a great social life. She had given up cigarettes in her thirties and was very proud of that, but also felt sure that this had contributed to her weight. At 46 Sarah found a lump in her breast, and had to have a radical mastectomy. She was devastated.

Having chemotherapy was horrendous and for Sarah, losing her hair was almost like losing her identity. She felt that she had had her youth stolen from her. She was also trying to cope with her two teenagers, and her weight ballooned. Comforting herself with high calorie snacks, within two years Sarah had developed diabetes.

This was her major wake-up call. The diabetes, luckily, responded quickly to diet, and Sarah lost four stone within one year. She started exercising regularly, and was thrilled when her hair grew back, thick and glossy, and her figure returned to its old self. Sarah quit drinking, following advice from her cancer nurse, and now only has one glass of wine a month, if that.

Sarah is now 66. This year, doctors did a follow-up bone scan and found one small spot signifying a return of the breast cancer in a bone in her chest. Sarah was frightened, but soon discovered that since her original cancer, 20 years ago, treatments have advanced considerably. The best thing is that she doesn't need chemotherapy. The bony metastasis is hormonally responsive, and Sarah is post-menopausal. Her oncologist has reassured her that she has had 20 great years since her first op, and thanks to a few smart lifestyle changes she will have many more years. She is responding to a mild anti-hormone treatment and the small spot on her bone is not increasing in size.

Sarah has had the test for the breast cancer gene, which wasn't available when she was first diagnosed, which found that she's negative. This is a huge relief to her, as she can be sure she will not have passed this disease on to her daughter or grandchildren.

Cancer in the family

There is a history of breast and ovarian cancer in my family. Am I at greater risk?

Consider genetic counselling, which accurately assesses your risk. You will be able to discuss the available options open to you. Some women who are found to be positive for the cancer gene opt to have their ovaries removed; some even opt to have their breasts removed. Counselling with full information is the most important help in making these types of decision.

My sister had breast cancer at 42. I am now 45, but have not been offered a mammogram. Why not?

Just because your sister has had cancer this does not automatically mean that you are at greater risk. Also, until recently, many oncologists and epidemiologists felt that mammography in younger women carries risks because of the radiation, which could cause more harm than good. In younger women, the breast tissue is denser so mammography is not as accurate, and there are more false positives. However, as the guidelines for screening are shifting internationally, current science seems to suggest that you do need a screening mammogram, and so you should discuss this with your doctor.

Another thing to do is to find out what sort of cancer your sister had. If she is still alive, ask her to have genetic testing. If she is no longer alive, you can quite reasonably request this test for yourself.

A diagnosis of cancer – empowering your body

- Reach out to other women friends, and ask them to help. Don't leave all the helping up to close family, who may be distressed.
- Develop a strategy for keeping up with work, hobbies, friendships and housework that takes into account tiredness, recovery time and rest.
- Consult with your employer regarding your rights and your sick leave scheme. Make financial plans for the future to remove stress about income. If you don't feel well enough to cope with these kinds of problems see if your union can help, if you have one.
- Accept that you'll be able to do a lot less than you used to, so learn to take your time, plan to do less, drop your standards. Get help in the house if possible. Many cancer support organizations offer help with housework, shopping, transport and other tasks. Save your energy for fun with family and friends.
- See a nutritionist and seek expert advice on your diet. Lose weight if you need to. Seek out cancer-fighting fruits and vegetables; if you are overweight, switching to a vegan diet makes a big difference and massively increases your intake of vitamins and antioxidants.
- Consider basing your diet on whole foods, macrobiotic (raw) foods, and soya-based foods, although discuss this with your oncologist first.
- Avoid alcohol from now on, except in very small amounts for special occasions. A target of one drink per week, or less, is your max.
- Try to avoid stress, tiredness, and situations that may lead to you picking up illness, such as late nights or travel.
- As soon as you have the energy, start to include some healing exercise in your life. Yoga, swimming, Pilates or walking can be gentle and relaxing and keep your body moving and strong, even if you are quite tired. As your treatment progresses, make sure that regular exercise is a daily habit in your life from now on.

My mother had cervical cancer, and my sister has cancer of the womb. Does this mean my risk is increased?

As far as doctors are currently aware, these are not cancers that can be identified with any particular gene. Although this is an unlucky family cluster, there is no reason to feel that your own risk is higher. Do have regular smears, however, and check for HPV. Although these cancers are not known to be genetically linked, the same social risk factors and lifestyle factors may 'run in families'.

My periods stopped abruptly when I began chemo for breast cancer in 1998. After one chemo session, I was in full menopause! I was 43 years old. I had noticed before this that my periods were heavier and painful. After this I began to gain weight and refocus my life as a person beyond reproduction. Sexual desire waned initially – then there was the chemo – afterwards, I certainly considered myself not very attractive. Maybe it was tied to breast cancer surgery, or just all rolled up into one! I realized that I had to reframe my identity. The biggest and most important decision I made was to spend more time with my women friends bonding. This is the one most powerful message I want to give to other women today.

8

Coping with forgetfulness and memory loss

The name of the author is the first to go
followed obediently by the title, the plot,
the heartbreaking conclusion, the entire novel,
which suddenly becomes one you have never read,
never even heard of.

These wonderful lines from the poem 'Forgetfulness' by American poet laureate Billy Collins might help to remind you that failing memory isn't an exclusively female problem! Forgetfulness is universal after middle age, and not just to humans. All animals need to keep learning and relearning, and the memory bank is only so large; it can only download so much software in a single lifetime. If you think of your brain as a very sophisticated and adaptable computer, then you'll find it easy to understand why after a certain saturation point in mid-life, new memories are competing for storage space among all the stuff you've accumulated all your life.

Memory and the brain

Neuroscientists are learning more and more about the brain, and one of the most important discoveries about our neurophysiology is that the brain is 'plastic'. This means that it is adaptable, throughout life. The actual material of the brain is a mass of neurones, long filament-like cells that receive signals from the environment, such as sound, light, smell. These sensory receptor neurone cells are threaded throughout the different areas of the brain, passing these stimulus messages back and over to other neurone cells, which can interpret their messages: cells in the language centre of the brain, in the emotional centre, in the memory retrieval centre and so on.

Memories are stored in the brain in a variety of ways, for example, as images, scents, emotions and sounds, and the marvellous thing is that we as humans have imagination in that we can conjure up these memories at will, creating our own images within our brains in order to create links with our past, in order to imagine the future, and in order to communicate ideas, beliefs and feelings of empathy. So, as a result of powerful emotional memories associated with your children, for example, based on a lifetime of sensory experiences, when you meet your child, you not only remember who he is, and what sort of relationship you have with him, you are always pleased to see him!

Another very important thing that our brain does for us in an adaptable way is enable us to learn new motor and cognitive skills throughout life. Although we may be born with a certain number of neurones, which give us some fairly basic skills such as walking, sucking, crying, avoidance of pain, we rapidly learn how to ride a bike, play a guitar, write with a pen and to use and interpret language, thanks to the adaptability of our neurone brain cells to take in new sensory information, interpret it and give a signal to motor neurones to operate certain muscles (such as in the voice box, larynx, fingers and legs) in a specific, task-oriented way. And, science now realizes, the ability of the brain to develop new neuronal pathways in order to learn new memories, or to up-skill new tasks, does not diminish throughout life in the healthy brain. New neuronal pathways do need to compete for space with the old: if you think about the analogy of the computer as a human brain, new software uploaded will compete with existing storage space. But, by constantly cleaning out old and unnecessary files you can create space for new information.

Menopause and the memory

If you think that your hormones are affecting your memory, you are not alone. Many women complain of struggling with memory shortly after menopause, and studies have linked memory difficulties or cognitive impairment with fading oestrogens. A lifetime of experience will tell you that your ability to concentrate can be affected by cyclical hormones. Many women report difficulty concentrating, for example, in the pre-menstrual period, or just after having a baby. But a hormonal explanation for memory loss is not adequate, nor is it conclusive.

The Alma Unit for Research on Ageing at Victoria University, Melbourne, Australia, studied the effect of ovarian hormone loss associated with menopause on cognitive function. The authors wanted to clarify the almost universal belief among the medical profession that failing oestrogen supplies to the brain after menopause were what caused memory loss. So, they decided to examine the effect of clear-cut, documented oestrogen depletion in two types of menopause: surgical and transitional. In other words, in women who had had their ovaries surgically removed, was lower oestrogen causing memory loss in the same way in which (it is assumed) women in natural menopause are forgetful because their ovaries are just getting old?

In order to eliminate any bias that the female patient might bring to the study, they decided to use female rats instead. They induced a 'natural' menopause in one group of rats, and in the other they removed the ovaries surgically, mimicking the sudden effects of menopause on a woman. Then they gave oestrogen to both groups of rats, and lo and behold, the oestrogen benefited cognition in the surgically menopausal rats but actually impaired cognition in the 'natural' menopausal rats. This made the authors of the study wake up to the possible harm that might be caused by slapping every post-menopausal and forgetful woman on to HRT. If we are to persist in blaming oestrogen for failing memory, we need to remember that oestrogen seems to behave differently in different groups of women, depending on how they came about their menopause. Thus, it's pretty fair to say that the understanding of the role of oestrogen in memory is pretty cloudy, at best.

In another study, in 2010, this time on real women, scientists at the University of California in Los Angeles wanted to find out what the effects of oestrogen were on a wide range of cognitive functions in post-menopausal women, and so they compared women who were currently using HRT with past users of HRT and those who had never used it. They looked at general cognitive, verbal, visual memories, delayed recall, attention, concentration and verbal comprehension skills among the three groups of women. They found no significant differences on verbal memories comparing never-users of HRT with past users. The authors therefore concluded that long-held beliefs regarding the usefulness of oestrogen supplements as a protective factor against cognitive decline in older women had to be questioned.

It's pretty clear that fluctuations in memory and depletion in cognitive function throughout middle and older age are multi-factorial. And that fluctuating hormones and ageing have a variety of associations throughout the female body, such as emotions, joint pain, sleeplessness, hot flushes, changes in body weight and mass, all of which impact on the way in which our brain perceives, interprets, creates, remembers and relates to the world.

In other words, memory and cognition is complex, and although fading oestrogens are associated with middle life, so is memory loss and fading cognitive efficiency. Therefore, although the two occur simultaneously, one is not, per se, causing the other.

So what's stopping me from remembering simple things?

New learnings come from a variety of stimuli, and are corrupted, enhanced or misinterpreted all the time as a result of confounding stimuli such as emotion, distraction, motivation, and physical health and well-being.

Think about the many other factors that your brain has to deal with, while you are learning something new, or reaching for a stored memory, which just wouldn't be an issue for a much younger person.

- Physical sensations: heat, cold, pain, feeling uncomfortable in your body.
- Sensory input: other people talking, competing noise, city traffic, the other job at hand like the fax you're waiting on, a ringing phone, the fading light, the ticking clock . . .
- Emotional/internal stimuli: self-awareness, tiredness, motivation, mood, anxiety, sorrow, worry, concern.
- Toxins such as alcohol or other drugs.

All these 'distractions' are present to your cognitive brain as a mature adult pretty much all the time, especially in middle age. You are probably still working, and/or managing a family. You are concerned about your own circumstances, about your changing body, your ability to work as hard as you used to, your physical appearance and your self-confidence. You are also taking on multiple concerns of others, at work, in friendships, in your family, extended or otherwise. You may have recently suffered loss, bereavement, divorce, employment, friendship; you may have had to move house, see a loved one suffer, or had to struggle with illness yourself.

Middle-aged women pretty much carry the world on their shoulders: right up there in the cognitive brain. If you do have any free mental space to learn an instrument, catch up on your French, or remember all the rivers of Africa in alphabetical order, it's a miracle.

What can I do to keep the show on the road?

Studies of memory retrieval, development of new memories (learning) and cognition (understanding) have shown that older people are perfectly capable of learning and memorizing new information and new tasks, as long as they have the desire to do so, and with the same stimuli to concentration, learning and memorizing that younger people are given.

Memory storage and retrieval

Memories are stored as information bits. That's all. In the analogy of the computer, it's as if you have a billion bytes of memories, which are stored as images, words, sounds, smells, emotions and so on. You can retrieve these, if your brain anatomy is not diseased and the particular memory neurons have not been destroyed. But, you need to know where to find them.

For most regular, day-to-day memories based on rote tasks, you just pick them up. You remember how to make a chicken curry, how to write an email, what to say when you answer the phone. You remember important details like your children's birthdays, your wedding anniversary, your blood pressure, your hair appointment – and you can't stop remembering that difficult meeting you had with your colleague yesterday! But it's the unimportant matters that get stuffed away in the attic of dull, unnecessary memories: the name of the actor who played Han Solo in *Star Wars*, the author of that lovely poem you liked in school, the name of those neighbours who lived down the road and moved to Seattle five years ago . . .

Making a memory retrievable means that you have to attach significance to it. This can be done by associating *something else* with the memory. So you mightn't remember the name of those neighbours who moved to Seattle, but if you have some time to yourself to think quietly about them and perhaps visualize them, you'll remember the name of their cat, the colour of their car, the job the wife did, the look of the teenage son – and then their name automatically comes to you.

Memorizing new information is a process whereby you take in external stimuli, such as words, sounds and sights, into your brain via the eyes and ears and send them through the visual cortex and auditory system into a variety of interpretive neurons (in the language centre, emotional decoding centre, and cerebral cortex) and then into your memory store in the parietal and temporal areas at the sides of your brain, to be filed away as images, sounds, emotions (such as the look of a word, the shape of something, colour, brightness and so on). So it requires a bit of neurological activity, efficient transmission of neurological messages between cells of different function, and an atmosphere that is conducive to the reception and perfect interpretation of data.

If you think about the breakdown of these events (receiving information, passing it on to the interpretive centres of the brain, and then storing it efficiently where it will make sense later on), there is a lot you can do, no matter where you are in life, to make this process as efficient as possible.

Lifelong learning

Research into patients with Alzheimer's, who have actively degenerating neuronal cells, has shown that playing computer games can enhance neuronal activities of existing healthy neurons, thus enhancing cognitive function and delaying dementia. Therefore, it is vitally important to keep instructing your brain with new learnings, and to keep experimenting with cognitive function to maximize your neuronal development and retention throughout life. You do need to apply yourself, avoid distraction, and to concentrate in order to learn. The good thing about learning is that it becomes a habit and the development of new neuronal pathways can only lead to more efficient use of your brain.

Learning and developing new knowledge and memories

It's a good idea to make sure that your learning environment is conducive to the intake of new information, and that this information is clear and understandable. Removing outside distractions such as noise, emotional distraction, and toxic pollutants such as alcohol or drugs, improves the accessibility of clear information to your brain. Concentrate. If you've been given new information, make an effort to pay attention to it. If you've just been told someone's name, make an effort to remember it. Don't be distracted.

If you have difficulty remembering names after an introduction, repeat the name and quickly remind yourself as you look at the person: 'His name is Peter.' When we meet someone new we often don't pay attention to their name, or attach it to their face in our memory system. You could attach some significance to the name: Peter the Great, Peter the Apostle, Peter Peter Pumpkin Eater . . . Or, think what animal, colour, or song the person reminds you of, which associates a visual or auditory memory with the name, making its retrieval easier later on.

Attach other mnemonics to new memories in order to be able to bring them to mind: colours, acronyms, rhymes and so on. In school we were taught to remember Boyle's Law of Physics, which is that at a constant temperature, the pressure of a gas is inversely proportional to its volume, by the mnemonic 'Boyle the kettle to make the T', evoking an image of a gas to make the T, temperature.

How to beat forgetfulness

If you're trying to remember some piece of information and it's just out of reach, and it's driving you crazy trying to bring it to mind, just stop. Research has shown that torturing yourself to retrieve a 'tip-of-the-tongue' memory causes that memory to be actually pushed further away and stored into insignificance. Memories are thought to be stored in loci, which contain a variety of aspects of the memory, images, words, emotions, sounds. Think instead about other aspects of the thing you can't remember: if it's the title of a film you saw once, visualize the actors, where you saw it, who you were with, the music and so on. This helps to retrieve the locus or context in which the memory is stored, revealing a whole pattern of memory from which the title can be retrieved.

List-making may help with boring, unmemorable tasks such as shopping, but it is not an aid to long-term remembering of new information. Instead, practise concentrating and paying attention to new information. De-clutter your head from distractions when you need to learn something new. Focus on the fact that you need to remember *and* attach significance to new information that's important.

Test yourself on new memories. When you really need to remember something for the long term, keep testing your recall. This is especially important for important passwords, PIN numbers, significant dates and so on.

Music is the most complex neurological activity we can do. Learning to read music and play an instrument automatically enhances new neuronal development throughout the cognitive brain, at any age.

Research into computer games has found that playing games enhances cognitive function, hand–eye coordination and fine motor activity. Chess, cards, golf, or any competitive game, encourages neuronal activity by removing distraction, focusing concentration, but most of all by rewarding targeted skill and learning acquisition.

The benefits of play

Adult life doesn't have to entail lack of fun! One of the main reasons that adults stop remembering, learning and being cognitively developed is because they don't *play*. Researchers into child psychology have understood for decades that children learn through play. The wonderful news is that this is by far the most efficient and effective way in which adults learn too.

Researchers at the University of East Carolina Psychophysiology Department studied the cognitive effects of video games on people over 50, and found major improvements to mental acuity as a result of playing games. Game players had an 87 per cent increase in cognitive response time (the speed at which they complete mental ability tasks) as well as a 215 per cent improvement to executive functioning (the frequency of completing those tasks correctly).

The researchers concluded that the 'active participation' required for playing a video game provides an opportunity for mental exercise that is much more beneficial than the passive mental activity of, say, watching television or listening to a lecture.

9

Improving disturbed sleep

Sleep is probably a menopausal woman's greatest luxury. Disturbed sleep affects at least 70 per cent of women during the climacteric, according to most studies, and many women report difficulty getting to sleep, or waking up during the night on five out of seven nights, As we get older, we tend to need less sleep, and all studies report shorter hours spent sleeping in both genders. But women are much more likely than men to report disturbed sleep as a problem. Most GP consultations regarding sleep are with women. Most sleeping pills are prescribed to women. The average time spent sleeping by healthy, non-menopausal adults is 8.3 hours per night. For menopausal women, the average time spent sleeping drops to 5.6 hours.

One study of 1,500 Scottish women aged 45–54, some of them menopausal, some post-menopausal, found that 40 per cent in the menopausal group complained of sleep problems. The good news is that this applied to only 20 per cent in the post-menopausal group. So sleep disturbance during menopause is likely to improve when the menopause is over.

A major problem associated with poor sleep is the fear of not being able to sleep. Days spent tired, cranky and unable to concentrate mean that your anxiety about a good night's sleep becomes worse. And a vicious cycle develops, because anxiety about being able to sleep is guaranteed to disturb your sleep anyway.

There are physical reasons for poor sleep, of course, such as hot flushes and night sweats, reported by up to 80 per cent of women. It's worthwhile developing the best possible sleep strategy during your climacteric years. If hot flushes are a problem at night, start by addressing these (see Chapter 3). Discuss your symptoms with your sleeping partner, and negotiate the possibility of opening windows or using lighter bed linen. Now is the time to invest in a larger bed, perhaps: a more luxurious mattress, extremely comfortable pillows.

What is sleep *for*?

Sleep is for healing. During sleep, the body secretes human growth hormone, from the pituitary gland, which is essential for tissue healing and repair.

There are two sorts of sleep: REM sleep and non-REM or deep sleep. REM stands for rapid eye movement, which we associate with dreams. Non-REM sleep alternates with REM sleep during a healthy, full night's sleep cycle, and we need these alternating waves of both kinds of sleep to feel refreshed.

Anxiety, stress, abuse, sadness, and other emotional disturbances cause overexcitation, leading to wakefulness. Wakefulness has varying effects on the normal balance of REM and non-REM sleep, thus affecting tissue repair of all the cells in the body.

Disturbed sleep, therefore, first affects the immune system, skin, gut and organs that need to heal the most regularly, pretty much on a daily basis. Ultimately, if sleep is inadequate for many days and weeks, end-organ damage can occur. Bone healing, cardiac output, blood pressure, and neurological activity can all be seriously affected by poor quality of sleep.

Menopause and disturbed sleep patterns

Normal healthy sleep is stimulated by darkness. During the day, exposure to light stimulates melatonin, which is known as the sleep hormone. Ageing after menopause is associated with reduced levels of melatonin, in response to tiredness or fatigue. Therefore, after menopause it becomes more and more important to stimulate your brain with daily *physical* fatigue, with intellectual or *cerebral* tiredness, *and* with daylight, in order to stimulate healing sleep.

During menopause, a pattern of deep, uninterrupted sleep may be replaced with a pattern of napping: wakening during the night, extreme tiredness the following day, requiring sleep after lunch. The wee small hours may be a time with which you start to become familiar. Pacing the house before dawn is a common complaint in menopausal women. Depending on what you do with your newly gained nocturnal life, this experience can be either distressing or fulfilling.

Nobody really knows why menopause is particularly associated with a sudden disturbance in sleep. Oestrogen therapy has had a variable effect on sleep: some women find it helps as it alleviates hot flushes, others find it no better than placebo. But the chances are that your sleep pattern will change during menopause, and you may have good and bad nights' sleep, wakening easily or needing to nod off during the day. The point is not to feel frustrated and angry about this change in sleep patterns, but to investigate ways of making your new sleep cycle work for you.

The important thing is to use your wakefulness productively, to develop a good sleep strategy for when you need to rest, and to enjoy a regular pattern of exercise, outdoor activity and cerebral stimulation, which help to regulate healing sleep.

Developing good sleep habits

Accepting that you may not always get a good night's sleep may free you from the constant anxiety that you 'can't get to sleep'. Talking to other women who have been through menopause will reassure you that you're not insane: we all need less sleep after middle age and we will develop variable patterns of sleep. Certain things are guaranteed to keep you awake, of course; the following are a few pointers to encourage the development of good sleep habits.

- Coffee, tea and cola-type drinks all contain caffeine which stimulates wakefulness, so have your last cuppa at lunchtime. Cutting back or removing caffeine-containing drinks from the diet altogether can't help but improve sleep. Camomile tea or hot milk at night has been found to help induce sleep.
- Watching television in the bedroom stimulates wakefulness; so does watching television at all in the two hours prior to attempting to sleep, or using a computer. Mobile phones and computers also emit microwave radiation in the bedroom, which is thought to prevent sleep. If you can remove all electronic equipment from the bedroom, this will undoubtedly improve your sleep.
- Make sure that you get at least an hour's outdoor activity during the day, preferably in bright daylight. Exercising before bedtime

has a variable effect: some find that it helps with sleep, others not. Be your own judge and experiment with your exercise routine.

- Many women find an evening yoga class helps considerably with sleep. If you can't manage this, a series of stretches to release muscle tension has been shown to help with sleep.
- Avoiding alcohol is one of the best sleep remedies. Enjoy your glass of wine with your weekend lunch rather than at night-time. Especially avoid alcohol with a heavy evening meal. Most menopausal women report that alcohol late at night, or with meals in the evening, result in disturbed sleep.
- Cigarettes tend to disturb sleep too.
- Clean your bedroom frequently. Vacuum and mop under the bed, removing all dust. Remove clutter from surfaces, preferably from your house altogether! Vacuum the curtains, or have them dry cleaned. Have fresh, clean bed linen regularly. Put all clothing away in cupboards, tidy and de-clutter wardrobes, keep all display items like lampshades scrupulously clean. Dust accumulates quickly in bedrooms and contains harmful faecal matter from mites, which can disturb sleep.
- According to the principles of feng shui, mirrors should be removed from the bedroom. Do your make-up and dressing in the bathroom instead. The foot of the bed should not point towards the door. Avoid plants, flowers and litter bins in the bedroom.
- Melatonin is a safe remedy, available over the counter in the USA, which is a gentle sleep aid (3 mg is the best dose; higher doses are reported, paradoxically, to cause wakefulness). It is only available on prescription in the UK but it is a lot safer than benzodiazepine or other sedative tranquillizing drugs, which cause side-effects and are addictive.
- Disturbed sleep can be a sign of depression, so if you are concerned about this, discuss your sleep problems with your doctor.

Sometimes you just can't help waking up during the night, or not getting to sleep when you want to. Use your wakeful early hours fruitfully, perhaps catching up on some work such as cooking, laundry, ironing and letter-writing – giving yourself some time off the next day to have a lovely long walk in the sunshine. The thing is not to become distressed because you are awake while others sleep.

Getting on top of stress

Write a prescription for yourself, telling you to put relaxation at the top of your agenda. Start by planning a stress-busting routine for every day; don't wait for all hell to break loose before you grab the yoga mat.

Keep a stress-source diary. When something upsets you, or causes you stress, make a note of what it was. You will begin to see a pattern. You may start to realize that you need to change a relationship, or even end a friendship. You may need to change your job. You may need to get rid of your mobile phone, or just delete all your emails! Finding the source of your main areas of stress will mean that you now have the power to do something about it.

Ask yourself, what am I putting up with that I could change? Letting go of the main areas of negative energy in your life will free you up to enjoy your menopausal years. You can and should slow down; take some time to reflect on the changes in your body and your mind. How can you let go of some of your old attachments, so as to live a more peaceful, simpler life?

Studies show that people with higher levels of perceived stress age more rapidly. Happy-go-lucky does seem to live longer. Cultivating acceptance can have a very positive effect on long-term stress and ageing. Studies of 'gratitude habits' have also shown that people who keep a gratitude diary are much more likely to feel well, happy, and be free from illness and stress.

Many of our stressors are in our environment: traffic fumes, toxic plastics and materials, unhealthy food and drugs. It's easy to get into a toxic cycle of feeling stressed, smoking or drinking in response to this, overeating, or eating unhealthy foods. If you are concerned about the effects that stress is having on your sleeping and ageing, think about ways in which you can 'detox' your life from these environmental stressors. Regular breaks in the countryside or spa treatments may help to detox your body from the struggle of city life. Detox juice diet days can calm your body and your mind, simply by focusing on your self and your health for a change.

In studies, women who took up regular meditation were able to reduce hot flushes at night by up to 60 per cent; up to 90 per cent of them were able to reduce or stop sleep medication. Meditation allows us to let go of judgements, let go of the past, and be present to the moment – to not sweat the small stuff. Try to develop a regular habit of daily meditation; start with just one minute, work up to five minutes, gradually building up to 20. Make your 20 minutes of meditation an appointment that you book with yourself which becomes sacred in your life.

Make positive affirmations at night-time, before you fall asleep. Use this time to think of the things you have achieved that day, the ways in which you have succeeded: what you are proud of, how well you have done. Think of what you are grateful for, this day. Think of those you love; visualize them one by one. If you find that worrying thoughts invade your space, promise yourself that you will give yourself time to worry tomorrow. Then, return to your positive affirmations.

Massage is a tried and trusted therapeutic intervention that promotes good sleep. See if you can persuade your partner or a family member to give you a massage before sleep; indulge in beautiful lavender-scented massage oils. Lavender oil can help to promote sleep, so add some drops to your evening bath, or dilute with almond carrier oil and massage into your own feet, neck, chest and abdomen before falling asleep.

Linda's story – a strategy for wakefulness

At the age of 46, Linda was in despair. When I met her she said she hadn't slept for more than three hours in a row for over two years, and was beginning to find that life was impossible to cope with. Her job as a senior business executive was very stressful, she had too much responsibility, and her relationship with her ex-partner was fraught with difficulty.

Linda sought advice from a life coach; following a good coaching session, she decided that the one thing she desperately had to improve in her life was sleep. She felt chronically exhausted and yet was living a high-energy life. She often had to travel for work, with very early starts, she always felt too tired to exercise, and tended to comfort eat; she drank a bottle of wine every night, just to wind down. Then every night she would lie awake for what felt like hours.

With help from her life coach, Linda realized that she needed a sleep strategy, a formula of behaviour and attitude that would guarantee sleep the moment she turned out the light. She started by asking people, other women she knew who were sleeping well, how they went about doing this.

'How do you *do* going to sleep?' was the question she asked. At first, many of her friends were puzzled. 'It just happens. I just fall asleep!' But Linda, as far as she was aware, hadn't 'fallen' asleep for years! She had to fight to get to sleep, every single night.

She realized that this was the clue, that it was this fight that was keeping her awake every night. One particular friend, who was able to sleep like a log, told her, 'I just fall asleep the moment my head hits the pillow.'

'Why?' Linda was desperate to know. 'What exactly goes through your head, the moment you hit the pillow, that makes you fall instantly asleep?'

'Well,' her friend replied, 'I remember that when I was at school I always had to stay up late to get my studying done. I was always exhausted but couldn't get into bed until I'd finished my school work. I used to look at the bed, longingly, almost crying with tiredness, desperate to go to sleep, but I'd work away until I'd finished, no matter how exhausted I was. And then I'd finally get into bed and it was heaven. Now, I get into bed and I just feel so grateful that I am in my bed. It's so wonderful to be lying down, with blankets, pillows, I don't care if I sleep or don't sleep!'

Linda immediately changed her attitude. That night as she lay awake, she didn't think about work, her problems with her ex-partner, or any other stresses that normally went on in her mind. Instead, she noticed how warm and cosy the duvet was, how comfortable the pillow underneath her tired neck, how peaceful her room, how quiet the house despite the sounds of the city outside, where other, much less fortunate people were still at work. She realized how grateful she was to be in bed! And fell asleep instantly.

She has had no sleep problems whatsoever since then.

A successful strategy for sleep

The difference between people who easily fall asleep and those who lie awake is just that: they are 'doing' two different things in bed.

It actually takes effort to lie awake at night, especially when you're tired. Research into people who lie awake has found that they are actually making a subconscious effort to stay awake. They are spending their time in bed worrying, thinking through to-do lists, problem-solving, feeling sad, mulling over old grievances, planning their next business deal, scheming, deciding important family matters. The point is that these are all actions, intense mental actions, which require wakefulness. Yet many of us save all these mental activities until bed-time, when they could so easily have been done during the day.

You may well feel that you can't 'stop' yourself from worrying once you get into your bed at night, but the truth is that if you are in bed doing something else, then you aren't doing your worrying. Learning how to 'do' sleep, rather than 'doing' wakefulness, isn't too difficult. It's a question of figuring out how you're doing wakefulness in the first place. And then, figure out how other people 'do' sleep and model them.

If, like Linda, you seem to have a strategy for 'wakefulness' rather than sleep, think about how you can change this.

- What is your night-time routine? Is it actually conducive to rest and sleep, or do you spend your evenings watching TV, drinking alcohol or cups of tea – in other words, disengaging your mind, and saving all your cerebral activity and problem-solving until bed-time?
- Mental activity – problem-solving and thinking – is very important and we all need to spend plenty of time each day thinking things through. Start by pencilling in an hour's thinking time during the day, perhaps during your daily walk or commute, as you take a bath, as you drive, while you cook supper. Or just lying down gazing at the sky.
- Don't be afraid to spend time during the day on your thinking by just staring into space, doodling, or playing a game. These are all

valuable ways of making sure that you get your thinking done in a more efficient way, at a time that is appropriate to you.

- You don't need to be stimulated by media all the time: switch off the radio and television and use the silence. Make time to do your thinking, worrying, deciding and mental activities while you peel potatoes, commute, exercise or mow the lawn.

- Think about how you do 'staying awake'. Do you lie there in a tense ball of wakefulness agonizing about all the work you have to do? Do you mull over insoluble problems, rather than enjoy the peace and comfort of your bed?

- As you get into bed, notice the comfort, cosiness and warmth as you lie down. Notice the pillow, supporting your weary head. The duvet, wrapping your aching body. The mattress, supporting your tired body as you fall asleep.

- If you sleep with someone, listen to their breathing beside you and think about how much you love that person and how grateful you are to sleep with them.

- Think about how thankful you are to be in bed, being this tired, while others are still at work. You've often been exhausted too, at work, perhaps driving late at night and unable to lie down. You've been on a plane, weary from travel, noisy airports, heavy luggage, and you have slept in a reclining chair, haven't you? You've been at work, desperate for an afternoon nap, and you would have lain down anywhere, even on the floor. You've slept on a train, on a bus, in the cinema. How often have you longed just to lie down and could not? And how wonderful it is, therefore, that you are in this bed right now . . . just lying here. How wonderful it is to be lying down . . . as you are now . . .

10

Looking forward to the future: staying healthy for life

Older women are the largest demographic in the world. If we can go back and redefine ourselves and become whole, this will create a cultural shift in the world and it will give an example to younger generations so that they can reconceive their own life span.

(Jane Fonda, at TEDxWomen 2011 in New York (www.TED.com))

Post-menopause: something to look forward to

In researching this book I talked to as many menopausal and post-menopausal women as I could. One thing always struck me. Menopause is no fun for any woman, just as puberty and adolescence is often the worst part of growing up. But afterwards, the fun is only just beginning! As post-adolescent adults we have this sudden realization that we can do whatever we want because our parents aren't in charge any more, we have an income and we are going places. The post-menopausal woman is going places too. She is wise, thoughtful, energized, adventurous and brave. She has lifelong friends and is open-minded to befriend new people too. She has family around her and yet can deal effectively with responsibility, preventing conflict and providing support when needed.

She knows how to spend time alone, cherishing her intellect and the space in which to be creative. She has travelled, and will travel more. She has seen over half a lifetime of experiences, people, places: she has lived through massively important moments in history. And, she has so much more ahead.

Change is inevitable, no matter what gender or age we are. The most important thing is to acknowledge the inevitability of change and to learn from it. Becoming older is a given, but becoming unhealthy or sick, developing pain, unhappiness or suffering are not inevitable. Illness will happen to all of us at some time in life, and for many women the early post-menopausal years are the most vulnerable in terms of loss of health. Life after menopause can be long and fruitful, if we are prepared to embrace it.

A normal healthy woman in Western Europe, Australia or North America can currently expect to live to be about 85 years old: and many of us who are now middle-aged will live well into our nineties. This is a remarkable shift in cultural expectations, compared to women at the beginning or even middle of the twentieth century. In the last 50–70 years therefore (the post-war and technology revolution years), our life expectance has pretty much doubled. We women can now expect to live 34 years longer than our grandparents expected to. This means that we are getting a whole extra adult lifetime. It's as if you've been put into a time machine and given a second chance – just when you expected to grow old and die, you got a whole new life. So, you have been given a second life, if you have just experienced menopause. The question now is, what are you going to do with it?

Yes, you have been given a whole different body. It's perhaps fatter, or slimmer, or slower, perhaps it sometimes hurts. But it's yours and you can treat it any way you want. You can work on it to change its shape, and you can choose to comfort it, nourish it, keep it strong.

Yes, you have been given a more mature mind. A mind that is so full of experiences, knowledge, memories and intellectual powers that it sometimes becomes completely overloaded. It needs to be cherished, recharged, rebooted, and it needs to be nurtured and treated with utmost respect. You can choose to make it magnificent.

Yes, you have been given the ability to love, to give to friends, to protect others who need you, to share your knowledge and wisdom with those who can use it. Yes, you have been given a deep and honest understanding of the world in which you live, as well as a ferocious curiosity that powers you forward every day to explore new ideas, take on exciting challenges and to make the most of every talent and ability you have. And yes, you have the ability to be a role model for others. To lead, share and collaborate with other women. To be proud of becoming an elder of a marvellous, haphazard, vulnerable, chaotic and powerfully driven society.

Mature women are now the largest demographic group in the world, and we are growing in number. We are powerful, strong, wise and we have everything to live for.

The next 30 or more years are a magnificent journey. And like every journey, they begin with a single list!

What you will need on your journey through your new life

1 A strategic-eating regime: your body is your life

- Make sure to eat five portions of fruit and vegetables a day.
- Every day eat something green, something purple or red, a handful of nuts or seeds: protect your body against cancer, ageing and heart disease.
- Every week eat oily fish: you need the omega fats for life.
- Eat less fat, and forget the refined carbs. Eat low GI carbs with every meal. Protect your bowels, heart, breasts, and waistline.
- Add vitamins whenever you can. Seek out meals that maximize vitamin content.
- Take low-fat dairy for calcium, plus supplements, and if you have osteopenia take calcium tablets plus vitamin D, every day.
- Eat small portions, at proper meals. Balance 50 per cent low GI carbs with 20 per cent protein and 30 per cent veg.
- Manage your weight carefully. Take your body size seriously: weigh yourself, check your BMI, measure your waist. Create weight and waist-size targets and stick to them.

2 A daily exercise habit: have you moved your body today?

Develop a programme of daily exercise for 30 minutes each day: timetable it, put it into your diary or schedule and stick to it. Do a weekly combination of aerobic exercise, weight-bearing exercise and stretching. A good strategy for the week during menopause and after might be: Monday – yoga class; Tuesday – swim for 30 minutes; Wednesday – weight training; Thursday – Pilates; Friday – walk for an hour; Satuday – weight training; Sunday – swim. You need to build muscle every day after menopause to prevent pain from arthritis, and to compensate bone loss from osteopenia and osteoporosis. This means taking weight training seriously, as well as aerobic exercise, which protects your heart (and brings you joy!).

3 Plenty of water to drink: protect your skin, kidneys and heart

- Skin thins and loses elasticity after menopause. Good hydration is essential for skincare as most of the water lost from our body comes through the skin, especially during sweating and hot flushes.
- For every cup of tea or coffee, drink two large glasses of water; the same goes for alcohol. A large jug left on the kitchen counter will help to remind you.
- Salt from food, which has a toxic effect on your heart and blood vessels, can be more quickly eliminated if you drink lots of water.

4 Find a doctor you like: trust her with your heart

- Heart disease is the number-one killer of post-menopausal women. Be disciplined about seeking regular medical check-ups, and protect your heart. Find a doctor or healer whom you admire and respect and take her advice.
- Have your blood pressure, cholesterol and urine checked every year, to screen for hypertension, hyper-cholesterolaemia and diabetes, especially if you have been overweight or smoked in the past, or have a family history of heart disease.
- Avoid smoking, alcohol and cardio-toxic foods; fried and salty foods are associated with high blood pressure.
- If you have been diagnosed with hypertension, immediately remove salt from your diet (never eat crisps, sausages, bacon, curry, takeaway foods and restaurant or ready-meals).
- Concentrate on whole foods, fruit and vegetables, small amounts of low-fat dairy, soya, nuts and raw seeds.
- If you quit smoking, remember that every day you don't smoke helps to protect your long-term health.
- Reduce your weight to a healthy BMI.
- If you have been diagnosed with hyper-cholesterolaemia, obesity and borderline diabetes, make immediate steps to try to manage these the drug-free way, before you decide or it becomes necessary to start taking medication. These are all caused by poor diet and therefore you *can* change that yourself.

- The damaging effects of poor diet, high cholesterol, salt and smoking on your heart and blood vessels can be difficult to reverse, the older you get. Attend to health problems immediately and take the advice your doctor gives you.
- Explore sources of stress in your life and try to eliminate these. You could discuss this with a life coach or other counsellor. Stress affects the heart; as your heart is the most important organ in your body, do not scrimp on the attention it deserves.
- Start practising mindfulness. Schedule a half-hour of 'silence' every day: be alone, without any stimulation, just listening to the silence.
- Learn to meditate. A life-long meditation habit promotes happiness, heals depression and improves hypertension and pain; it can also positively affect outcomes of cancer and other chronic diseases.
- Make a regular appointment with your 'self'. Every day, stop for a moment and ask yourself, 'How *am* I?'

5 Spend time with friends: they can support you and make you happy

One of the strongest messages that came across to me as I spoke to older women is the enormous benefit of the bonds that many senior women develop throughout life. If you have not taken time to nurture friendships with other women, start by doing that right now. Nobody needs to be alone.

- Start to make a special effort now to prioritize friendship and close relationships, rather than career, money or personal 'success'. Become a member of a club, find like-minded friendships and exercise your skills, exploring interests and learning.
- Do not be fooled into thinking that you are too busy now to have hobbies or interests outside work and immediate family, and that you will join that choir, French class or sailing club when you retire and have more time. It may become more difficult to have the courage to do so by the time you get around to it. Think ahead and have a strategy for developing your mind throughout your life, enhancing your intellectual interests and enjoying your social life.

- Learn to enjoy spending time alone. Develop your creativity. Pencil in a time to be creative every week: painting, drawing, gardening, writing, dressmaking, playing an instrument. Work, rest, and always, always make the time to play.
- Develop a strategy for joy. What makes you happy? *Where* are you happy? How do you know when you are happy? What is happiness *for*? Answering these simple questions will tell you a lot about your values, who you are, and where you want to go in life!

6 Cherish your relationship: keep it strong

Take time to continue to nurture your relationship. After menopause, most women experience less frequent episodes of sexual desire, but are still very excited by sex, lovemaking and intimacy. Studies by pharmaceutical companies, searching for a medicine that would work as a 'female Viagra', have found that no such medicine is necessary in women! The reason is that after menopause, we are still quite easily aroused, and do not experience 'impotence' as men do. However, throughout life women are not excited in the same way as men are, simply by the glimpse of a stocking or a naughty garage calendar. We require loving, intimacy and emotional arousal before we can experience orgasm, and therefore although we will experience sexual pleasure throughout life, at any age we will only experience this after desirable foreplay.

While many couples have less frequent sex after menopause, this is not an issue for most people. We can make sure to enjoy frequent exchanges of affection and maintain a strong friendship, as well as ensuring that sexual experiences, whether infrequent or rare, are made more pleasurable by romance, loving emotions and foreplay. Vaginal lubricant from the chemist can make the experience even more exciting.

Growing older: being yourself

For many older women, the years after the age of 60 are the happiest in their lives. What do these women have in common? Most will say that they feel that they are 'themselves', that the years have brought a sense of no longer feeling as though 'others' come first: others' lives, others' values, politics, emotions, power games. Jane Fonda gave an inspiring talk at an event organized by TED (Technology, Entertainment, Design – a non-profit organization devoted to 'Ideas Worth Spreading'). In her talk, she described her own feelings about growing older as a journey in which she decided to look back at her past and get to know herself again. She learned to forgive herself, to realize that her failures were not her own fault, and that she was just the same person that she'd always been: it's just that when she was younger, she forgot to be feisty, forgot to be herself. Like most younger women, she was constantly distracted by the approval of others.

One of the strongest messages I've received from talking to older women is that after middle age, we begin a new confidence. We can stop worrying about what others think of us all the time. We can start, many of us for the first time in our lives, to 'be' ourselves. And, in being ourselves, we can become role models for others.

Who are you going to become, in your new, adult life?

What I noticed most during menopause was the acceleration of the ageing process: a deterioration of energy, muscle tone, skin and hair. Sometimes a sudden rise of body temperature. But these changes did not distress me much. I did become bothered because I attributed to the menopause certain symptoms (sleeplessness, irritability, feelings of chest constriction, palpitations, loss of libido) which I now believe were merely coincidental and caused by anxieties about teenage children, grief over deaths in the family, a decrease in self-confidence and heightened aware-ness of mortality. What I'd say to other women is try to find a way of reconciling yourself to growing older and don't let the negative image of old women in our society cast a shadow over the rest of your life. (*Penny*)

Please think of menopause as a part of the natural cycle of life. Be proud to be an 'elder' in your community and promote inclusiveness among women, not competitiveness. Boost your daughters and sons, don't mourn your youth.

Set a good example of authentically living a meaningful life in the face of change. Try new things! Disclose your feelings to other women. Don't isolate yourself! (*Florence, age 56*)

I can't remember noticing any immediate physical differences and this was probably because my life changed dramatically at the age of 54 when I opted for early retirement and embarked on a VSO placement in Zanzibar. So, physical changes that took place at that time I put down to coping with my new environment – I lost weight, was more active, took some time to adjust to the heat. My hair thinned due to medication to prevent malaria, but when I stopped taking this medication my hair improved! (*Helen, age 70*)

I love being older. I love my life. I am 79 years old, a widow and I have had a stroke and have arthritis in my knee, but other than that I'm fine. The stroke didn't really affect me much and I can drive, which is the most important thing. I am blessed with wonderful friends who are clever, interesting and kind. I know all my neighbours and I can trust them, which is very necessary as I am away a lot.

My life is a bit too busy sometimes but I don't mind. Every week I go to classes because I love learning, I'm always doing adult education. At the moment I'm studying horticulture, which is very exciting. I travel twice a year to visit my daughters in America and England. I always have to try very hard to get them out walking as my great love in life is hill-walking, and they don't exercise much! I've climbed so many mountains!

The best thing about retiring from my job as an accounts manager is that I got to do another degree and so I graduated from university at the age of 70. I was really proud of that. I did a degree in Music and Spanish. That's what I love most in life, singing and music. What I'd tell menopausal women is, you're young! You're so young. You don't realize it but the best is definitely to come. I'm looking forward to another few decades, anyway. (*Elaine*)

Index